KU-014-608

The New Diary of a

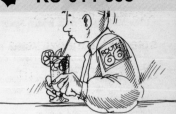

TEENAGE HEALTH FREAK

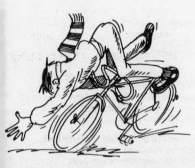

Aidan Macfarlane
and
Ann McPherson

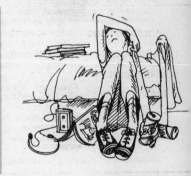

Illustrated by John Astrop

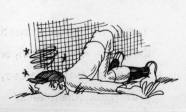

Oxford   New York
OXFORD UNIVERSITY PRESS

Oxford University Press, Walton Street, Oxford OX2 6DP

Oxford New York
Athens Auckland Bangkok Bogota Bombay
Buenos Aires Calcutta Cape Town Dar es Salaam Delhi
Florence Hong Kong Istanbul Karachi
Kuala Lumpur Madras Madrid Melbourne
Mexico City Nairobi Paris Singapore
Taipei Tokyo Toronto

and associated companies in
Berlin Ibadan

Oxford is a trade mark of Oxford University Press

First edition, under the title The Diary of a Teenage Health Freak,
first published 1987 as an Oxford University Press paperback
Second edition, under the title The New Diary of a Teenage Health Freak,
first published as an Oxford University Press paperback 1996

British Library Cataloguing in Publication Data
Data available

ISBN 0-19-286182-4

10 9 8 7 6 5 4 3 2

Printed in Great Britain by
Mackays of Chatham plc
Chatham, Kent

The New Diary of a Teenage Health Freak

Pete Payne, aged 14, suddenly discovers one day that he suffers from hypochondriasis—that he is, in other words, a confirmed health freak.

For the next year he proceeds to confide to his diary such fascinating medical details as he is able to glean from any available source—including extracts from his 13-year-old sister's diary, which he sneaks a look at whenever he gets the chance.

His wide-ranging research, including much first-hand experience, extends to subjects as diverse as acne, warts, alcohol, drugs, headaches, depression, accidents, sex, diet, and generally surviving life with his parents and two sisters.

When his diary was originally revealed to an unsuspecting world the result was astonishing: teenagers piled out from behind the bike sheds to grab it from their friends; relieved teachers and startled parents were to be seen surreptitiously checking facts in well-thumbed copies. In response to international pressure Pete has now divulged the complete, unabridged, totally unexpurgated version, with no details spared—for other teenagers who want to know but are too embarrassed to ask, for parents who know some of it but are too embarrassed to answer, and for teachers who know most of it but don't have time to explain.

AIDAN MACFARLANE is the director of the National Adolescent and Student Health Unit and a Consultant Paediatrician in Oxford.

ANN McPHERSON is a general practitioner with extensive experience of young people and their problems.

As well as *The New Diary of A Teenage Health Freak* and its sequel *The Diary of the Other Health Freak*, their other books include *Mum I Feel Funny* (which won the Times Education Supplement Information Book Award), *Me and My Mates*, *The Virgin Now Boarding*, and, most recently, *Fresher Pressure*—an amusing and informative survival guide for students.

JOHN ASTROP has written and illustrated many children's books, including *My Secret File*, *Not Now Dear!*, *After All We've Done!* and *Little Stars*.

'Spiffing, first class, splendid, excellent and altogether BRILLIANT!'

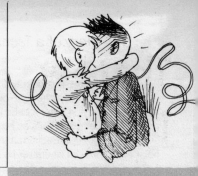

'hilariously funny . . . tells us the things my friends and I have always wanted to know, without the embarrassing idea of having to ask someone.'

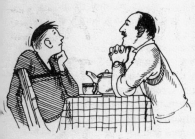

'It was so good that I couldn't put it down: I read it until two in the morning and couldn't get up in time to do my paper round! . . . essential for all teenagers and parents'

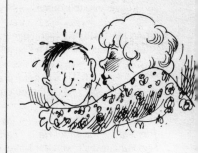

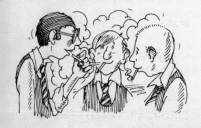

'I am glad someone at last ha the guts to write out funny or rude things you wouldn't say in the public supermarket'

Acknowledgements

Much of the material in the original book was provided by the 4th-year pupils at Lord Williams's, Cheney and Peers Upper Schools in Oxfordshire. We would like to thank them and their overworked and underpaid teachers who kindly and bravely prevented chaos whilst the pupils answered our questionnaires and wrote for us about their health and their problems. For additions to the Second Edition we would like to thank Isis Middle School, Ravenspark Academy, Kate Roberts, Alice Coulter, Laura Harris, Alice Maclennan, Michael and Niall Paulin, and many other teachers and teenagers—too numerous to mention—who responded so positively when we approached them for suggestions on updating the text.

We would also like to thank Marny Leech for her invaluable help and advice.

This book was also much aided and abetted by our children, Beth, Gus, Magnus, Sam, Tess and Tamara, and their friends—who often surprised us and sometimes horrified us by their revelations concerning sex, drugs, alcohol, divorce and much else besides.

On their behalf, and because of their huge admiration for another diary writer, we wrote more in hope than expectation to Sue Townsend to ask whether Adrian Mole could possibly take time off coping with Pandora to give us an opinion on what Pete Payne had to say. Very, very many thanks to them both for their response.

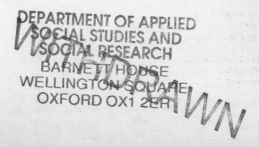

Contents

Book Review by Adrian Mole ix

About this diary's writer xi

1. How I Learnt I Was a Hypochondriac 1

2. Crashing the Pain Barrier on a Bike 7

3. Feeling Fed Up 15

4. School Gets Busted, Pupil on Dope 24

5. Has Susie Started Yet? 33

6. My own 'Life Changes', but they Take a Long Time 41

7. Learning to Live with my Zits 49

8. Sally's Sex Life Goes Wrong 54

9. Susie Gets Hayfever 56

10. My First Fag Nearly Kills Me 64

11. Pains, Sprains, and Wheezes 72

12. Sick, Sick, Sick, or the Summer Holidays 81

13. Future Fears 90

14. Little and Large 102

15. Wart-Hogs and Odious Odours from Orifices 115

16. And so to Jaws 3 123

17. Days off School 129

18. Four Eyes 138

19. Drunken Desires 144

Index 153

Book Review by Adrian Mole

At last! A book for hypochondriacs and sophisticated teenagers like myself! I read it through in one all-night sitting, and found (by the time the horrible birds started their early-morning screeching) that I had 110 ailments; 15 serious, 10 fatal.

I immediately went to see Doctor Grey in his tatty surgery. He looked through the book and then settled down to read it. After half an hour his irate receptionist stormed in and said, 'Doctor Grey, you've got fifteen patients waiting.' Doctor Grey put the book down and said, 'I must buy a copy, get out Mole you are 100 per cent fit. Stop wasting my invaluable time.'

On re-reading the book I was struck by the amount of down-to-earth frankness about sex. My neurosis about this subject, especially about the length of my 'thing', has now diminished. Here are all the answers to the questions I've never dared to ask.

I remember asking my father how babies got out of women's 'stomachs', I was four at the time. My father blushed bright red, lit a foul cigarette, poured himself a Scotch, scratched his head, pulled his trousers up AND NEVER GOT ROUND TO ANSWERING. Talk about a coward! I tottered into the kitchen, dragging my teddy behind me, and asked my mother. She said, 'What are you, a pervert?' She believed in using grown-up language to small children. So for years I thought women had zips on their stomachs. In fact, I blush to confess, I was eleven years of age before Barry Kent told me about THE FACTS OF LIFE. We were sitting on a canal bank. Shortly afterwards he pushed me *into* the canal—I didn't mind too much, I needed cooling down because I'd got hot and bothered. He spared *no* details.

I wouldn't mind meeting the author of this book. We've got a lot in common. (Though of course I am a genius, and an intellectual, and he's not.) We've both got a lousy family life, delicate health and disfiguring pustules.

I've left my copy of this book on the kitchen table next to the ashtray, so my mother and father are bound to see it. If only it had been published years ago. I might have been saved much personal anguish.

Pandora, the love of my life, is coming round to read up on, and I quote, 'Girl-related health situations.' She's been suffering from Pre-Menstrual Tension (or, to be more accurate, everyone around her has been suffering). At certain times of the month she changes into a monster; Doctor Frankenstein's creation looks like Noddy in comparison to Pandora in one of her rages.

Yes, this is the book for my generation. Teenage Hypochondriacs of the world unite! We have nothing to lose but our health!

A. Mole

About this diary's writer

GENERAL INFORMATION

Name Peter H. (daren't tell you the rest) Payne.
Nickname 'Know It All Pete'.
Date of Birth 17 December 1980.
Age 14 years and 1 month—year 9 at school.
Born according to Mum, half-way down the
   corridor at the hospital, on the way to the
   labour room.
Address 18 Clifton Road, Hawsley, London.
Hobbies picking my nose, watching telly, playing Nintendo,
   worrying about myself, teasing my younger sister, annoying
   people by being a 'know all', collecting medical facts, reading
   photographic magazines, having accidents.
Heroes Harrison Ford, Nelson Mandela, myself, Sam's dad,
   Adrian Mole, whoever it was discovered penicillin but I can't
   remember, Pamela Anderson.
What I'll be when I grow up myself, a famous scientist, very
   rich, and very very attractive to girls.
Personality at the moment shy, awkward, unattractive to girls,
   afraid of life, shirker at washing up, tease (especially of
   Susie), bad at sport; but enjoy helping old ladies cross roads,
   doing my homework before watching telly (except when *Match
   of the Day* is on), making witty comments and being original.
Worries catching AIDS, GCSEs, growing up and being
   unemployed.

PHYSICAL MAKE UP

Sex male and becoming more so.
Height five feet and four inches against my doorpost using
   Mum's measuring tape.
Weight 58 kilos but ate a big supper.
Hair colour brown.
Eye colour brown to match.
Distinguishing marks the whole of me but especially the brown
   birthmark on my bum.

MY MOTHER

Name Jane Elspeth Margret.
Date of Birth June 1953 but can't remember date.
Age 35 for the last six years.
Job part-time in building society, cook, cleaner, clothes washer, general neighbourhood 'do gooder', doctor to all of us, looking after Dad, worrying about us all.
Weight chubby.
Hair colour brown.
Eye colour green with flecks.
Distinguishing marks her laugh, like a sick hyena.
Personality noses into my private life all the time, makes me be nice to stupid relations, doesn't take any notice when I have sleeping problems etc. and just says 'you'll get over it', is always saying 'have you done your homework?', but is cuddly, a good listener, and doesn't bother me about my room the way Sam's mum does.

MY FATHER

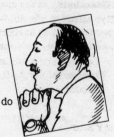

Name Anthony Tobias.
Date of Birth don't know.
Age nobody knows.
Job kills tiny beasties in people's houses. It's called 'pest control' which is what I do to my sister Susie.
Weight expanding.
Hair receding—what's left of it.
Eye colour can't remember.
Distinguishing marks awful moustache.
Personality funny, good mechanic, won't stop smoking secretly, always talking politics, knows about a lot of things.

MY OLDER SISTER

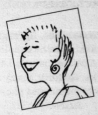

Name Sally (and Beatrix—TOP SECRET).
Date of Birth keep forgetting.
Age 17.
Weight a state secret.
Hair colour changes all the time.
Eye colour blue.
Distinguishing marks two bouncy ones in front.
Personality worse 'know all' than me, bossy, and will do almost
    anything for money which she's saving up to buy a motorbike
    with.
Favourite Music Meat Loaf, Michael Jackson, Ace of Base.

MY YOUNGER SISTER

Name Susie Jane (lucky her—they'd run out of
    awful names).
Date of Birth tells us about six times a day—16
    January 1982.
Age 12 years and 11 months.
Hair colour mousy.
Eye colour mousy too—like the rest of her.
Distinguishing marks none.
Personality worries about what her friends will think of her
    family, enjoys shopping, giggles, doesn't obey my orders, and
    overreacts on purpose when I tell her off, especially if Mum's
    around.

MY BROTHER

Unfortunately Mum and Dad never gave me one.

MY BEST FRIEND

Name Sam Sproggs.
Sex says he's male.
Age claims he's 14. Most of the time behaves like he's 4.
Personality crazy about bicycles, attractive to girls but ignores them, tries to be original but isn't, gets more pocket money than me.

ROMANTIC ATTACHMENTS

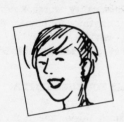

Name Cilla Jeffs.
Sex yes, if she'll let me.
Age 14.
Where she lives not saying.
Why I like her just do.

PETS

Type cat (Sally's) which would starve to death if Mum didn't feed her.
Name Bovril.
Age 14 demented months and losing all her hair.

MY HOUSE

Semi-detached with more bays than the South Coast. Metal round the windows like every other house for miles around. Three bedrooms and a shoe-box for Susie. Pink tiles in the bathroom. Fitted carpets everywhere. Hairs on Mum's suite where the cat's been. Kitchen fixtures care of Dad, so not quite finished yet.

MY ROOM

'IN and OUT' message board on the outside of the door, and paper skeleton on the inside. Bed with all my old clothes down the back. Pooh Bear one million times over on my bedcover. Dad's yellow paint over bumpy wallpaper, picture of aeroplane by me, covered with Pamela Anderson picture from Sally's *More*. Books and comics everywhere ranging from *Asterix* to Stephen Hawking's *A Brief History of Time*—looks good but I haven't got past the first page.

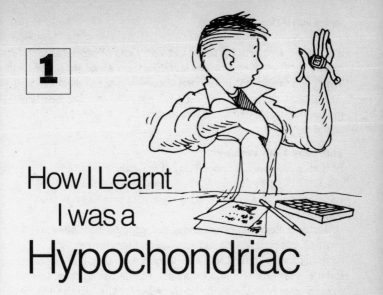

How I Learnt
I was a
Hypochondriac

Wednesday 11th January

The biology teacher set me off today. Going on and on about how wonderful and efficient our heart is, giving 80 beats per minute, which makes 3 billion pumps during a whole lifetime. Estimated mine's already done 80 times 60 times 24 times 365 times 14 = 588,672,000 beats. (My calculator ran out of space—need a better one.) Worried about all this work my heart's already done; felt sure it would never last out. Asked Mrs Smellie whether I was likely to have a heart attack in the afternoon's cross-country run. After all, Grandad died of a heart attack dashing for a bus last year. Know he was 80 but was dead worried it might run in the family. Smellie said not to be stupid. Exercise is good for the heart and helps stop heart attacks when we're older—just like NOT smoking does. She never misses a chance of telling us how wonderful NOT smoking is. Said the odds of me dying from a heart attack at my age are less than one in a million anyway—less likely than winning the National Lottery. Next worry was Mrs Smellie remarking that I was actually suffering from a bad attack of 'hypochondriasis'. Sounds much worse—suppose I die of it? Asked what the symptoms were, but got nowhere. She just told me to 'look it up'. Might just get around to it, if I don't die tonight.

Thursday 12th January

Still alive. Managed a second day of my diary! New Year's resolution was to start on 1st January—only ten days late! It was reading Adrian Mole and my mum stopping nagging that inspired me.

Nothing much happened today except my sister, Susie, kept on at Mum about having Kate as well as Mary for her 13th birthday party. I hate them all—they're so boring. Mary's the sixth 'best friend' she's had in a week. Mum's taking them to some dismal Walt Disney film on Monday for the fourth time. Really babyish but it's the only thing on. I'm going to go to Sam's instead.

Haven't died from hypochondriasis disease yet—perhaps it's not as serious as I thought. Sam's dad will know—he's an expert.

Saturday 14th January

This hypochondriasis thing is beginning to worry me. Sneaked into the school library at lunch-time yesterday and got the dictionary down, when in comes old glass-eyes Slogs, the school swot, wanting to know what I was looking up. Didn't want him to realize I have a dread disease . . . might be catching and everybody would avoid me. Looked up 'EROGENOUS' instead. Glass-eyes insisted he knew what it meant, but went pink behind his pebble lenses when I read out loud (for the benefit of the sex maniac illiterates present, and for the effect on Miss Bellows, the 60-year-old music teacher, slumped half-asleep over her music score): 'Areas of the body causing sexual excitement, such as nipples, ear lobes, and the inside of the thighs.'

Helped Dad mend the car today. Wish we had a BMW 560 series like Sam's dad instead of our tenth-hand pile of rust called a Vauxhall Cavalier Estate, but it's better than having a posho Volvo Estate like Randy Jo's dad. It's just that ours won't start in this slushy weather. Sounds as though it's dying of lung cancer—a bit like Dad coughing in the mornings after a forty-a-day binge. We had to get it started to go for lunch with Aunty Pam tomorrow. Wished Dad would give it the kiss of death instead of trying to make it work.

Met Sam later and cycled over to watch his team play football. You'd have thought I was Scott, off to the Antarctic, the way Mum insisted I wrap up—'so you won't catch cold'. Embarrassing and hardly streamlined, even on my old bike. Sam's got a Titanium-framed mountain bike, with a Shimano XTR group set and Maric rims, a Panaracer Smoke on the front, and a Panaracer Dart on the rear, to say nothing of the Pace RC 35 forks—which he won't let me try. Says I'll bust it. All this doesn't matter too much to me, except his mum lets him go out dressed in his sleek 'Tour de France' black Lycra—makes me feel a real jerk.

Sam's team won but the goalkeeper broke a leg, and will be out for the rest of the season. Heard the crack as it went. Left before the visiting thugs (don't know why they call them fans) were let loose from their cages. Not only am I a coward, but I hate violence. Cycled home at top speed to help my heart pump the way it should (estimate I am near the 600 million mark now). Slowed down again in case it made the hypochondriasis disease worse.

Sam came to tea and dribbled jam from his doughnut all over the sofa of the new three-piece suite. Had to lick it off, cat hairs and all. Sam loves coming to tea with us. At his house he's never allowed to have white bread, chips, bacon and egg, tomato sauce, chocolate biscuits, or coke. Maybe Mum's not so bad after all; or maybe I have this hypochondriasis thing because I eat so badly.

Susie's a pain when Sam's around—always trying to talk to

3

him and show off, even trying to join in conversations about football and bicycles, as if SHE knows anything about them. She used to hate my friends, but now she's suddenly all over them—is this what the books call 'PUBERTY'? Couldn't she just stick to girls? Don't fancy a lesbian for a sister, but what's that make Sam and me?

Argument about telly with Mum. Lost as usual. The same old things—it strains your eyes, makes them red, makes you bad tempered, gives you a headache, makes you violent, turns you into a sex maniac (I told her I already was one, which didn't help much). She went on and on. I don't get enough sleep, I always watch rubbish—and anyway, I'd already watched the football on Sky sports and would be watching Match of the Day. She said Dad should never have got that satellite dish as she hates the way it looks. She'd prefer to be like Sam's parents who refuse to have Murdoch beamed into their front room. No support from Susie on this as it was football. It would've been different if Sam had been around, which he is most of the time—watching Sky! No support from Dad as his team lost—bloody traitor.

Still worrying about THE DISEASE.

Sunday 15th January
Forced up by Mum at 12 o'clock. Still furious with her about the telly. Such a hypocrite—she watches The Big Breakfast Show. Mum and Dad just don't understand. First they say I need a lot of sleep and then they complain when I stay in bed late. Their problem is that they can't make up their minds.

Car sick on journey to Aunty Pam's. Susie read all the way. How can SHE do it without feeling sick? It's not fair. Mum wouldn't let me sit in the front and no one wanted the window open because of the cold—till I said I was about to throw up.

Aunty Pam's place smells awful—dog shit, cat pee, beer on Uncle Bob's breath, Aunty Pam kissing me with all that sickly powder and perfume! There should be a law against grown-ups kissing children over 12. I wonder what you can catch from kissing and bad smells. Always knew I couldn't stand Uncle Bob;

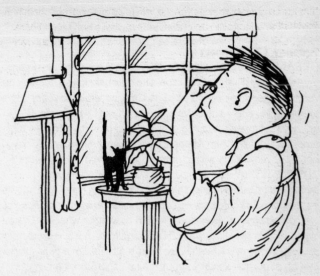

now I know why. First thing he said was, 'I notice you've got a bit of a moustache, young man.' As if you could call the growth on my upper lip a moustache, and anyhow I've devoted a lot of effort to NOT noticing it. Susie and Mum laughed and I made things worse by blushing. Bad enough having this hypochondriasis, without my other blemishes being pointed out.

Asked Susie whether any of her friends had hypochondriasis. She said, yes, lots—and what I actually was, was a hypochondriac. Bloody know all, worse than me, but didn't dare admit I didn't know what it meant.

Monday 16th January
Went round to Sam's. His dad's a medical expert doing research with animals into something called 'immunology'. Wonder if he read all about medical things when he was my age? Hoped he'd reveal all about 'hypochondriasis'—he seems to know about everything, but he was away at a conference. Sam says that's where he goes whenever he needs a rest.

Susie had her friends for a birthday supper after their film while I was out. Kate's invited Susie for next holidays. Good.

Tuesday 17th January

GREAT DAY. Got to school early. Amazed everybody including myself. Arrived just as Whitton, the caretaker, was opening up. Very surprised to see ME at that time, normally catches me sneaking in behind the bicycle sheds after the bell's gone. I usually find myself tripping over a crowd of sixth-formers all smoking. Told Whitton I'd some work to do in the library. Took down the dictionary with clammy palms—and here we were. 'HYDROPHOBIA—an aversion to water, especially as a symptom of rabies.' Help, this was something else I had got as I hate baths. 'HYPNOSIS—state like sleep in which subject acts only on external suggestion.' I began to wonder whether I had everything in the dictionary. 'HYPOCHONDRIASIS—abnormal anxiety about one's health.' So that's all it is. I'm a person who has an abnormal anxiety about his health and not a terrible disease.

What a relief—though I have to admit that there IS just a bit of this in me, because thinking back, in a way I was a little disappointed there was nothing seriously wrong with me. I had begun to imagine myself lying in hospital with piles of chocolates and grapes, my family and friends by my bedside: Mum in anguish for not letting me watch more telly, Dad promising to give up cigarettes, and Sam really sorry he hadn't let me ride his fantastic bike. Can see how a hypochondriac's life could be a happy one.

Thursday 19th January

News still full of the earthquake. Glad I'm not there.

2

Crashing the Pain Barrier on a Bike

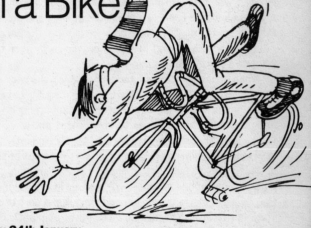

Tuesday 24th January

Exhausted by not having THE DISEASE. Given up on my diary writing resolution.

Wednesday 1st February

Have had a major accident and am stuck indoors, so may as well start writing my diary again.

Last Saturday started OK. Sam called and we went off on our bikes to visit a friend of ours called Joanna, as Sam had a record she wanted to tape. They disappeared upstairs leaving me feeling a right prat. Then Nick, another friend of ours, arrived and took my bike, so for a laugh I rode Sam's round the close. As I am fairly short in the leg I couldn't really handle it, and going down the steep hill I suddenly couldn't find the brakes. At the bottom was a row of houses and a sharp left turn. Still searching for the brakes, I slid on some ice and hit the kerb. As I flew over the handlebars I heard something going CRACK—a sound I'd heard before not long ago—and that was it.

Next thing I remember was being in the ambulance. The driver and his mate were laughing and telling jokes. I couldn't understand what had happened. My Levi 501s were ripped, my left arm was blown up in a plastic bag so I couldn't move it, and my head hurt like hell. Everything was coming and going, and I felt sick and faint. There was no siren blaring. The paramedics said they only used that in real emergencies, or when they wanted a cup of tea in a hurry!

When we finally stopped and they opened the back doors there was Mum, crying, and Dad, white-faced. Dad started swearing and telling me what a bloody stupid thing it was to do, and had I done it on purpose to worry them, and why didn't I think about these things before I did them? Honestly, grown-ups! Mum told him to shut up. I wanted to get out of the ambulance by myself, just to show I was all right, but the paramedics pushed me back, wrapped me in a red blanket like I was 80 or something, and carried me out in a sort of chair. They said I'd broken my arm and the blown-up plastic bag was to keep it still and stop it hurting. Mum clutched my good hand and Dad dragged along behind, muttering about Sam being furious over the scratches on his bike.

They wheeled me into a little white room and put me on a hard bed. Nobody seemed to bother much about me, though I could hear someone saying something outside about a tetanus injection. Mum had to go out and ask if I could have something for the pain—and came back saying that the nurse was sorry but they were busy. At last a nurse came and shoved a thermometer in my mouth and held my wrist. If she wasn't as pretty as the nurses on telly she was certainly as nice. She helped me take my torn jeans off. My poor legs looked white and were covered in grazes. My heart nearly stopped when I thought she was going to take off my underpants too.

A man came in and asked me questions about the accident, and some silly things like what day was it and who was the Prime Minister? He looked into my eyes with a light, stuck pins into my legs to see if I could feel, hit my ankles, and then examined EVERY last bit of me. Finally felt brave enough to ask what it was all about. He said it was to make sure I hadn't done any damage to my brain—like being concussed. Turns out that this is like bruising your brain, but it gets all right in the end. The 'silly questions' were to make sure it was functioning OK.

Nobody seemed to have actually DONE anything yet, then a lady came in and started examining me again. Wondered just how far SHE was going to go. She explained that the man was a medical student and learning, and that she was the actual doctor and was going to arrange for my head to be X-rayed to make sure none of my skull bones were broken, and my arm because she was sure that was broken. More waiting and nothing being done. Began to want to be home in my own bed.

The lady doctor showed me the X-rays and said I was lucky not to have dented my skull and damaged my brain. She said she couldn't understand why people didn't wear crash helmets when cycling, because 200 cyclists are killed and 24,000 injured in England and Wales each year. If I was thinking of getting a motorcycle in the future, I would HAVE to wear one. But even so, 469 motorcyclists are killed on the roads each year, and 26,000 injured. To emphasize the point, she said that she spent most of every day putting together people who had had accidents, and that in any one year:

> 1 in every 24 motorcycle riders
> 1 in every 107 car drivers

are killed or involved in an accident. It doesn't even seem safe to walk around, as 1,300 pedestrians are killed and 49,000 injured each year. All this doesn't even include other types of accidents like drowning which kills over 200 children a year, or the 2 million-plus people treated by the hospital for home accidents each year. HELP!

Asked the doctor if SHE wore a crash helmet when she bicycled. She went pink and didn't answer. Mum gave me one of her special looks and said I seemed to be getting better. Dad went back to work and Mum stayed while they put sloppy wet white bandages on my arm which made it warm. Bit by bit the bandages grew hard and smooth and I was left with a lovely shiny white plaster for my friends to write on. This stops the ends of my broken bones moving so that they can heal properly. Said they might replace it with a fibreglass one later.

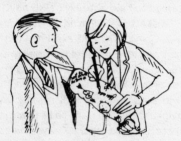

Just as I thought everyone was finished there was one more thing—an anti-tetanus injection. The dirt in the cuts on my knee might have contained tetanus bacteria. This could give me lockjaw, which is spasm of the muscles of your body, not just your jaw, and can easily kill you. Mum said I had last had the injection when I was 5 but that it only protects you against tetanus for about ten years and then you need it again. I said I'd had a jab at school last term, but apparently that was against measles or something.

Because I'd been knocked out, they said I might have to stay in hospital for the night. This frightened me at first, but then I thought it might be quite fun, especially if all my friends came to see me with presents. I'd missed out on this with my hypochondriasis disease. However, I was allowed home with my mum because everything seemed all right, but with instructions that she should bring me back if I began to throw up, had a bad headache, saw double, or became drowsy because of the knock on my head. They also said to come back if the fingers of my broken arm became numb, swelled up, or became white or blue. Sounded nasty but didn't happen. The last four days have been boring—no fun playing Nintendo with one arm—which is why I am writing all this.

Nobody's been to see me except Sam—to complain about his bike. Though he did manage to ask me how I felt. Then he went on about how some girl called Beth in our class was soft on him. Dad said that I've suffered enough and that he'd pay for the repairs to Sam's bike. He can be great sometimes. Susie and Sally have been sympathetic too. If I haven't many friends, I suppose having sisters is better than nothing.

Thursday 2nd February

Up early to catch the bus—first day back in school. Was the centre of attention for five seconds while everyone (except Cilla) defaced my plaster with graffiti, some of which I feel embarrassed to be carrying around in public. Pity I haven't got one of those new lightweight fibreglass ones yet.

Had to sit out and work during the sports periods. Don't usually like sport but now I can't do it, I feel left out. Mr Jones, the sports teacher, is orgasmic about exercise and says we could be almost mega-fit if we did at least 20-minutes exercise three times a week, enough to make us sweat. He said that as I had nothing better to do I'd better be the form representative for the school magazine and get some articles for the next edition.

When I finally got the chance to tell my mates about my accident (with a few embellishments about my bravery and my attractiveness to the nurses) I found I could hardly get a word in. Turned out everyone thought they'd had a worse accident than me and they were going to tell me about it whatever happened. Got fed up and told them to write about their troubles for the school magazine.

Thursday 9th February

A whole week without writing. Too exhausted by my one-handed
efforts at home and in school. Lucky I'm not into GCSEs yet. All
the teachers have stopped making allowances for the fact
that I'm a cripple. Stories for magazine coming in well. The
things my form mates seem to get up to . . .

'I was playing 40–40 up the shop with my sister and a friend about
four years ago. I ran out across the road to get 'in' and a big red bus
hit me just as it was going to stop. My sister went to get my mum.
She came running out and I was just running round and round. The
doctor came and he got me and my mum to the hospital. I slept in
the hospital for the night. I just had a bit of concussion. I went home
next day.'

Jan

'I broke my nose right across the bridge. I was standing with my
brother and he was shaking the rain off his hair and I walked into
him and broke my nose. It gave me headaches, and a purple and
very embarrassing nose. I went to the hospital and first they said I
would have to wait till the swelling went down. Then they sent me to
the ENT clinic. No one was really sympathetic about it.'

Tim

'About three years ago I was hoovering in the hallway. A piece of
paper would not go up the hoover so I pushed it in with a knife, and
my fingers got sucked in and all cut up. Also, when I was about 10, I
was sitting on the sink in the bathroom and it fell off the wall and I
hit my eye and it was all bleeding.'

Jo

'I've had at least three accidents but none of them serious. The first
was when I got kicked by my pony at a show, but I wasn't hurt badly,
only bruised and slightly sore. Then I was bitten by another pony
while I was doing up his girth. This hurt more than when I was
kicked, because it cut the skin and I was bleeding. Another accident
was when I fell off and got dragged along the road. I was riding a
small pony, taking her back to the field, when two girls came running
down the road and startled her and she darted under a low branch
and knocked me off. I clung on to the reins and she dragged me
along for about 100 yards. I hurt all of one side and I still have the
scars.'

Sharon

'Me and another girl went for a walk by this railway line. There were three boys chucking stones and one big stone landed on my head. They rushed me to hospital. I lost three pints of blood and had to have sixteen stitches—six inside and ten outside. They had to give me five injections in my head to make the skin numb when they stitched me up. I had to stay in hospital overnight and when my parents came and told me the news I started crying, so the doctors let me go home. My sister was there when the stone was in my head and my cousin, who pulled the stone out, said she could see my skull bone. The doctors and my parents thought I was going to die because if the cut had split any more I would have been gone. Now every time I see people throwing stones I run indoors and I think that that fear will always stay with me. If anyone hits me round my head or touches it I go mad and throw out at them.'

Liz

'My last injury was just over a month ago when I went ice skating for the first time. I can roller skate but I had been told by my friends that it was harder because you slip over everywhere. I went skating with some of my friends but when I got on to the ice I was very frightened because when I tried to move I slipped over. Then everything was going great until a boy behind me pushed me over and I went crashing into the side of the rink. As I did this I put my hand on the floor. Some boy who was standing next to me skated over my fingers. I started crying because I was in a great deal of pain. My friends saw me and helped me off the rink. My fingers were pouring with blood and all the skin was ripped back and my nail was cracked and bruised. After the accident I decided never to go skating again—but I did.'

Judy

'My last injury was when I electrocuted my right hand. It happened when I turned on this lamp. I had been using nail varnish to make the bulb red. The effect of the burn on me was that I couldn't write for a month. I had to go to hospital as it was an electric burn which apparently is much worse. I had to have plastic surgery and the skin was taken from the outer part of my other hand. I was in hospital for three days.'

Dave

'When I was 10 I put my hand through a window. A chunk of skin came out and I was rushed to hospital. I was told I had to have a skin graft. I didn't know what that was then, and now I wish I hadn't had it because I'm still scarred and I think that I will be scarred for life. It is very embarrassing because the skin was taken from the smooth surface of my arm, and you can still see it.'   *Kate*

'I was on a bike coming down a hill. I was with a friend who was in front of me. A car was in front of my friend. He went right into the door as it opened and flew over the door and hit his head as he landed. I went up the back of him and went over the handlebars, swearing like anything at the driver. I came down with my leg underneath my bike, and my other leg twisted round the handlebars and the brake cable. The bloke got out of his car and said my friend was all right and I told him what I thought of him. My friend got up and was slightly concussed but not much. I got hold of his bike and carried it home and then went off to the police station with my dad and my friend's dad. It has confirmed my feelings about people who do not look properly before opening their car doors.'   *Tony*

'I had an accident on my bike and twisted my bollocks and had to have sixty stitches in my bollock bag . . .'

Anon (I think it's Randy Jo)

I made sure this last one didn't get to Mr Jones. I think this guy is just trying to boast. I put it in here because I think it's what's referred to as a 'tall story'.

Friday 10th February
Nose bleed after sitting on the lav picking. Blood everywhere. Thought I was dying again.

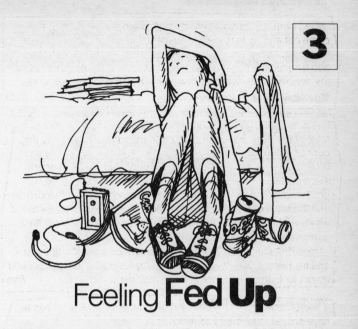

3

Feeling **Fed Up**

Wednesday 15th February

Big argument between Mum and Dad last night. Something to do with camping in the summer, and Gran, and how she'd insist on bringing her spare false teeth in a plastic bag, and not wanting to have the police searching for them again. Seemed OK this morning, but they wouldn't tell us about it. When I asked, was told by Dad not to pick up fag ends. That's rich coming from someone who pretends he's given up smoking. Back cycling to school again after two weeks on the bus. Glad to get rid of the cast but still scared by what they said at the hospital about my fingers going numb, or blue, as my hand still hurt. Everyone crowded round at school and Cilla, who I really like, wanted to touch my arm. It looks all white and pathetic out of its cast.

Usual chaos in French. Miss Dunlop is hopeless at keeping order. Sam and I sat at the back discussing summer plans for cycling and camping. Told him about Gran. Caught chatting—my first detention tomorrow, so maybe they'll all realize I'm not such a swot after all. Didn't get any Valentines yesterday. Sad, but at least I didn't send any. Sam got two, of course.

Tuesday 21st February

Mum and Dad getting at one another again this evening. Sally made it worse by saying she was going to be out late. Mum said she should ask, not tell, and what about that last bit of A-level course work? Sally flounced out saying that all her friends were allowed to stay out late, even on weekdays. Her parting shot was that she was not only old enough to get married, but also old enough to have a baby. Could see that shook Mum rigid. Beat a hasty retreat to my diary. Heard Sally coming in early, slamming the front door meaningfully.

Seems that Mum's got more control over Sally than over Bovril, the cat, who's out all night waking the neighbourhood with her sex life.

Wednesday 22nd February

Worried as woke with a headache. In such a state nearly mistook Mum's sleeping tablets for paracetamol, and forgot my maths book. Was late meeting Sam who was furious. Both late for school. Sam disappeared with other friends at break, and I had no one to talk to. Finally had to stay on for my detention. Not only bored with all my work at school but couldn't even be bothered to play Nintendo.

Thursday 23rd February

Sally spent hours in the bathroom tarting herself up for Mike, her latest boyfriend, while everyone else hung around waiting. Susie's been moaning about having no friends. Kate's gone off and found a new best friend—don't blame her. Susie yelled at me for not passing the sugar at tea-time. She's too fat to have it anyway. Turns out Beth's asked Sam to the cinema on Friday, and what's more he's going. Thought I was going with him. He seems to like Beth more than me and, much as I want to, I'm too shy to ask Cilla. Maybe I'm gay because I'd rather go with Sam.

Friday 24th February

Pouring with rain—got soaked going to school. Both Mum and my maths teacher asked me if I had got out of bed the wrong side. Felt exhausted and had a headache all day, and was still fed up with the thought of not going to the film.

Then came the BIG bust up. Like Bosnia but on a domestic scale. I spilt some tea by mistake. Susie said it was on purpose because it was her turn to clear and wash up, and that I had to wipe it up. Didn't see why I should as it was HER turn. She made a face and stomped to the kitchen with a pile of dishes. So I spilt her tea, and when she came back told her now she had something of her own to clear up. She tried to hit me. I caught and twisted her arm. She fell and hit the table and the milk bottle fell and smashed on the floor. At this point Mum reappeared looking as black as thunder. Told her it was all Susie's fault and Susie, lying as usual, said it was all mine. Mum threw a washing-up cloth at Susie and a brush at me, telling us to get on with clearing it up. Then she walked out in a real strop.

Immediately Susie slopped milk all over my new trainers, whispering, 'I hate you', so told her she was a real pain and no wonder Kate didn't like her any more. As I said it, I was aware, with terrible certainty and delighted fear, that this would provoke violence. She hit me on the arm with her milk-sodden tea towel, so I screamed and collapsed (unhurt) on the floor clutching my arm and shouting she'd broken it again, but actually cutting myself accidentally on the broken glass on the floor.

At that instant both Mum and Dad appeared—Mum at one door speechless with rage, and Dad at the other, fresh from beastie bashing, equally speechless. Mum recovered first, yelling, 'BOTH TO BED—NOW.' Dad blurted out, 'Do what your mother says or I'll get in the United Nations peacekeeping force.' I cried, 'But I'm bleeding,' and Susie said, 'But it was all his fault, why do you always pick on ME?' 'BED,' Mum screamed, so, deliberately dripping blood all up the stairs, I stamped up to

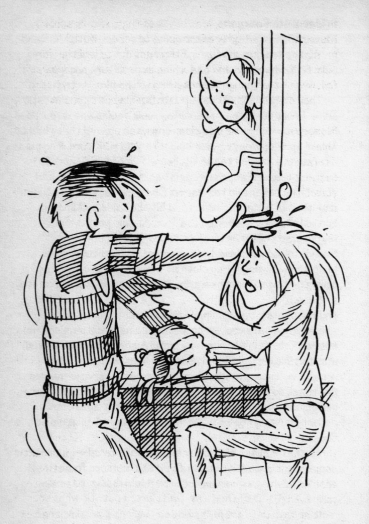

my room, slamming the door. Lay listening to Susie sobbing. Maybe 'feeling fed up' is infectious.

What seemed hours later, Sally came up to fetch us for supper. In Susie's room the sobbing immediately began again, followed by a shout of, 'No—leave me alone, everybody hates me.' In my worst whiney voice I recited as loud as I could:

'Nobody likes me, everybody hates me,
Think I'll eat some worms.
Big fat juicy ones,
Slip slap slimy ones,
Watch them squiggle and squirm.
Bite their heads off,
Suck their guts out,
Throw their skins away.
Everybody wonders why I live on three fat worms a day.'

Sally shouted at me to shut up. When I stopped I heard her say to Susie, much to my surprise, 'No, they don't hate you. We all think you're great, including Pete.' Lies, lies, lies.

Supper was a dead silent affair. Had neither the energy nor the nerve to reject my kidneys and green beans—even though I didn't feel hungry. Dad made one or two of his feeble jokes which disappeared into the generally shitty atmosphere without a ripple. Came straight up after supper to write this. Sometimes writing about things seems to make them better.

10 p.m. Thought I had finished for the day—but couldn't sleep for Mum and Dad shouting at one another and the throbbing of my cut. The argument seemed to start again with something about Gran coming on holiday, but the battlefield soon broadened to become more bloody and make less sense than even Susie and me.

It appeared Dad never gave Mum any support looking after us, never did any cooking, washing up or cleaning, always forgot her birthday and for that matter Valentine's Day, never put the lav seat down after peeing, never fed the cat, never washed the bath after himself, spent the whole of some nights with a headache, never wiped his feet, always left oily bits of the car all over the sitting-room sofa, and was always indulging our materialistic needs and never considering hers.

Dad, in Mum's pauses, claimed that she always left the car with no petrol in, was illogical, never appreciated the fact that he came shopping with her, always got the pages of the newspaper muddled up, never put the top back on the toothpaste and, worst of all, us children were becoming just like her . . . and so it went on.

Suddenly felt absolutely miserable and really worried. Did this mean that Mum and Dad were going to get divorced? It would be all my fault. I had, I had to admit, started it all, when I was feeling fed up. If Mum and Dad separated life wouldn't be worth living. We'd be passed backwards and forwards like Charles and Di's kids.

I wasn't tired any more. I had to talk to somebody, anybody, about it all. I crept along to Susie's room but she wasn't there, so tried Sally's and there were Sally and Susie curled up in bed together chatting. I collapsed on the floor with a sigh, aware of the silence that had descended downstairs.

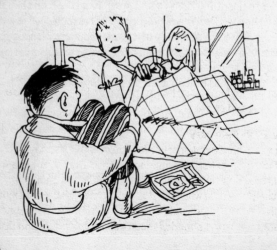

Sally then started doing her 'Mum' act. 'Don't worry, it's not yours or Susie's fault. Grown-ups often have rows. I'm amazed you haven't heard Mum and Dad before. You two are not the only ones to quarrel, you know. An occasional row is a normal part of life and Mum and Dad yelling doesn't mean they don't love each other. You have to know someone really well to be able to love them AND know how to hurt them too! Mike and I have terrible rows sometimes, about the silliest things. But I think it's better than bottling things up, like Uncle Bob and Aunty Pam have been doing for the last twenty-five years. There's nothing like a good row for clearing the air. You wait and see tomorrow.'

Tried telling Sally how awful I felt, and she really seemed to know what I meant. She even put a plaster on my cut.

Saturday 25th February

Woke this morning knowing it was going to be a better day—and it has been. First Dad made breakfast! Mum was very appreciative. Dad even kissed Mum in front of us. Mum said that I looked tired and I rather tentatively joked that I hadn't been able to sleep last night for all the noise. 'Oh,' Mum said, 'I hope you weren't listening to our "discussion" last night.' We all laughed, and I added that next time Susie and I had a 'discussion', please would they not interfere. Dad said not to be cheeky.

Sam came round later to complain that Beth had brought two friends with her to the cinema and that the girls had all sat together and expected him to buy them ice-creams. He's gone off girls and stayed for supper.

Monday 27th February

Nothing much happened on Sunday, but at school today a group of my friends were discussing parents. Mat's parents are divorced. They had terrible rows all the time, threw things at one another, and then when his dad finally left, no one told him the truth—his mum just said that he'd gone off for a holiday. This scared me, but it sounded much worse than Mum and Dad.

Mat said that even if he wished his mum and dad were still together, it was more peaceful now.

When I got home, Sally had left one of her magazines on my bed. It had an article by some child psychiatrist about teenagers feeling depressed.

Moods and Depression in Teenagers

Sometimes it is difficult to tell the difference between being fed up and being depressed. One tends to merge with the other. Some people see being depressed as being very, very fed up. However, we all feel fed up sometimes, and perhaps even occasionally a bit depressed. Luckily few of us suffer from severe depression. Many of the things which make us moody can seem much worse, and indeed almost insurmountable, if we are already depressed.

Listed below are some of the things which may cause *you* to feel this way:

* feeling very lonely or unsure of yourself
* a friend committing suicide
* your parents separating or getting divorced
* your parents having rows or arguments all the time
* feeling unable to manage your life
* one of your parents getting very depressed
* being seriously ill yourself or your parents getting ill
* having rows with your close friends
* problems and worries with your work
* your parents always expecting you to be wonderful.

If several of these problems occur together, you may feel it is impossible to cope and even wonder whether it is worth while going on living. If this happens, help and treatment are available. It's much better to try to talk to somebody about it rather than keep it all to yourself. The best person is somebody YOU find it easy to talk to. It may be your best friend, your mother or father, sister or brother, teacher, doctor, priest or vicar, aunt or a sympathetic friend.

It is sometimes difficult to recognize exactly when being fed up becomes being depressed, but this list might help:

* feelings of complete hopelessness and helplessness
* feeling that everything in the future is going to be bad
* feeling that the smallest task is impossible
* being very self-critical over a long time, so that you think nothing you do is ever any good
* feelings of continued tiredness over days or weeks
* being unable to sleep for many nights on end, and waking up early in the morning when this is not normal for you
* frequent headaches and/or tummy pains for which there is no obvious cause
* loss of appetite with loss of weight, or compulsive eating
* feelings of being cut off from everyone around you, including family and friends
* work suddenly seeming much more difficult to do
* staying away from school or running away from home.

None of these things by themselves, or just lasting for a few hours, or a day, mean you are seriously depressed. However, it is when one or more of them occur over several weeks that this may be depression and you should then get help. It is not nice being depressed. It is like an illness and needs to be treated.

If you think one of your friends is depressed, try to get them to talk to you about how they feel. If they are feeling *really* bad, you ought to tell someone else about it—maybe your parents. Sometimes your friends may find it easier to talk to *your* parents than their own. Otherwise discuss it with a teacher or someone else you trust.

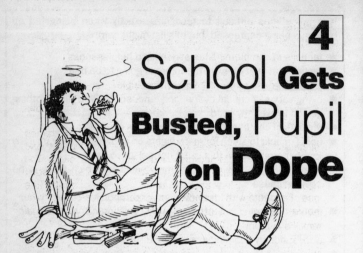

4 School Gets Busted, Pupil on Dope

Monday 6th March

Decided I'm not depressed, but can now recognize a teacher or two who is. At least my headaches have gone.

Tuesday 7th March

Found a book about sex and puberty in my room—wonder how it got there?

Wednesday 8th March

Real excitement. Reporters, police everywhere asking us questions. A geek called Smith in the upper sixth, who usually spends all his time swanking and bullying fifty-kilo weaklings like myself, has been pushing hash to year 9. Mr Rogers found some poor kid throwing up behind the bicycle shed. Heavy interrogation by Mum when I got back. She'd heard it on the local radio news. Had he pushed it on me? Had I ever tried it? Had any of my friends? By the time she'd finished I was convinced my whole form was on heroin. Anyhow I know Mum takes a sleeping tablet now and again. Told her she'd better watch it or she'd become an addict herself.

Susie's ill with diarrhoea. Hope I don't catch it.

Thursday 9th March

Out at seven among the joggers and the dog shit to get the local newspaper. Fame at last. There it all was:

Seventeen-year-old Pupil Pushes Dope

A sixth-former at Wendles Secondary School was arrested yesterday for allegedly selling cannabis to junior pupils. He blamed his friends for getting him hooked on it. 'First time I had it was at a friend's house on a Saturday evening. It had been all planned beforehand to get me stoned, which I was rather angry about at first. But in the end I was excited about taking it, rather than frightened or anything. At first it was just like smoking a cigarette but getting a pleasant effect as well. I kept laughing. It was like being drunk without the sick feeling. I only smoked it when I was offered it at big parties. Then I met somebody who said they could get the stuff real easy. My friends started coming to me for it. Then this person started getting heavy. He wanted me to start using other things, but I refused. I know what other drugs do to people. No way would I inject

anything. I think that's disgusting.'

Police Inspector James said, 'That's the way these kids often get hooked. The "hard" drug pushers start them on something like cannabis and then say, "Why don't you just sniff a bit of this?" or "Just put a bit of this in your drink", and before they know it, they're hooked on heroin, cocaine or amphetamines. It only takes two weeks of heroin, two to three times a week, to be addicted.'

Mr MacIntosh, the headmaster, said he was naturally horrified, and wanted to reassure parents that nothing like this had occurred in the school before. An earnest-looking Year 9 pupil said he thought it was disgusting. If alcohol and tobacco had been discovered now they'd also have been made illegal, and it was high time they banned smoking in the teachers' common room. Smoking and alcohol were just another kind of drug.

It was me! That's what I had said to the bloke—and they had put it in the paper!

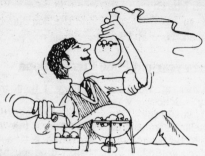

Friday 10th March

Rumours everywhere. LSD being sold over the counter in the school shop. An amphetamine factory in the chemistry labs (half the school was in there today trying to find out if it was true). Mr MacIntosh gave a talk at assembly. Dead silence as he started. 'It has come to my notice (hardly surprising—as it has been in the paper and on the radio!) that certain elements (did he mean us?) are bringing the school into disrepute by their activities. The staff have instructions to look out for any evidence of the evil practice of drug taking having spread. I've already suspended one boy. Other suspensions will follow. Do not get the idea that we are soft on drugs.'

All in all, he was pretty serious about it. A feeling of excitement built up. Little groups huddled in corners whispering to one another and staring suspiciously at any passing sixth-former. Poor Sam was even hauled up in front of the head for using his inhaler. Didn't tell Cilla about my quote in the paper. Maybe one day she will read my diary and appreciate my genius.

Sunday 12th March

Boring weekend. No good films on, invasion of Susie's friends. Tried watching TV non-stop, but got fed up. Maybe I'll try cannabis after all.

Tuesday 14th March

Two men in faded blue jeans, who'd been hanging around the

school for the last couple of days looking like sex maniacs or local flashers, were actually policemen from the drugs squad. Had to miss biology for their talk. Worth it though. Scared me shitless, as they probably intended.

They started by saying there is no single reason why teenagers like us take drugs. Most of us will be offered them at some time or other, probably at parties or in a pub, usually by someone we know, and most of us will say no. But some of us will try them, from curiosity, boredom or because friends are doing it. Here are the facts they gave us.

The police can stop and search anyone they suspect of carrying drugs. In the United Kingdom last year there were about 50,000 drug offenders of whom 25,000 were cautioned, 12,000 fined and 5,000 jailed. The maximum prison sentence for supplying other people with heroin, cocaine or lysergic acid (LSD) is 'life', and for using any of these drugs—fourteen years. The maximum prison sentence for supplying other people with cannabis, cannabis resin or amphetamines is ten years, and for using them—five years.

With a bit of luck, 'spliffy' Sapen Smith might get put away for ten years. (Wonder if you can take your A levels in prison?)

They then explained that when people talk about drugs they might mean drugs which are medicines and help you—like penicillin, insulin, and paracetamol. But even medicines have to be used properly. If you take too much of a medicine, or the wrong kind, this can be harmful, and they gave insulin as an example. People with diabetes, when their body doesn't make enough insulin, get sick because the amount of sugar in their blood gets really high. They have to inject themselves with artificial insulin, but if they inject too much then the sugar in their blood gets too low and they can pass out, because the brain needs some sugar from the blood to keep it going. However, lots of drugs AREN'T medicines—the ones you get arrested for if you take them. These can do harm and with some of them, once you start taking them, it is very difficult to stop.

They then made us write down all the reasons we could think of why any of us would want to take illegal drugs. I think I must be a natural addict as I'd got the longest list:

* to feel big and hard
* to feel excited about doing something illegal
* to know what it's like
* to be like other people who are taking drugs
* to rebel and be different from everyone else
* to get my friends to admire me
* to upset my parents
* to forget about my problems, like not knowing how to tell Cilla I fancy her
* because it's fun.

The police looked at my list for so long, I was convinced they thought I was already an addict.

They gave us this leaflet called *Know Your Drug Scene*, and said it was better to have at least some idea of what you were getting into if you were using illegal stuff than to be ignorant.

Cannabis
So what is all this cannabis stuff?
Cannabis comes from the hemp plant. It contains something called THC (tetrahydrocannabinols) which is the chemical that has the effect.

It has more names than most people have had hot dinners, including dope, pot, weed, grass, hash, marijuana, blow, draw, rocky, black, leb, gear, puff.

It normally either looks like dried-up grass, or comes in a hard block.

It is usually smoked but can also be eaten.

What happens when you take it?
If you smoke cannabis, it starts having an effect after a few minutes and the effects can last up to three hours; but if you have a

bad time with it, it can take much longer to wear off. It can have very different effects on different people:

* you may feel great—happy, relaxed, talkative, and giggly
* you may feel as if you are much more aware of what's going on around you
* you may feel anxious, confused, withdrawn, depressed, and that everyone is getting at you
* you may feel a combination of these things.

So why all the fuss?

If you use a lot:

* you begin to . . . oh, yeah . . . sort of . . . umh . . . forget things
* you lose your, what's it called? That thing . . . um, er . . . concentration
* this can give you trouble with your schoolwork and your social life
* in fact, you can become a real 'dope head'.

OK, so that doesn't sound so bad

Well—there's more. If you tend to get a bit depressed or anxious anyhow, then there's a form of cannabis called skunk (because it stinks) which makes you sleepless, bad tempered, and not nice to know at all.

And the real problem?

The police—it is illegal to possess cannabis, to use it, or to supply it. If you're found with it, you may just get a caution or a fine (but don't count on it) or you may get a prison sentence—up to five years for possession or ten years for supplying.

In fact, the majority of people in Great Britain on drug charges are there because of cannabis. Most people don't know that.

WHAT YOU MOST CERTAINLY WILL GET IS A POLICE RECORD WHICH COULD RUIN YOUR CHANCES OF GETTING A JOB OR GOING ABROAD.

Both policemen admitted it was just as well one habit didn't always lead to another. They'd be on the big H by now, as they both smoked like chimneys. I'm still determined not to get hooked on even nicotine. Perhaps I can get some money out of Dad for not smoking, like Sam's dad's promised him.

Wonder if all these facts might make someone actually want to try drugs? Doubt it though, especially after what was to come . . . the bad effects of the other drugs.

The leaflet went on to say that drugs like **amphetamines**, which are also called speed, uppers, whizz and billy (crazy names), can stop you sleeping. They make you restless, they make you sweat, feel dizzy and very anxious, and then you collapse exhausted and feeling depressed.

Ecstasy did not sound ecstatic at all, but it seems it's on its way out now. It was mainly used at raves, as it makes the music sound better and people able to dance longer, but quite a few people have died when using it. Nobody knows exactly how much damage it can cause, but there are real worries about it harming your brain—so if I took some I would never be able to understand Stephen Hawking!

The real nasties are heroin, cocaine, and some sort of chemical alternative called 'crack'—which is the worst for getting addicted. **Heroin** is also called junk, H, gear, smack or brown. People using it regularly get called 'the living dead', with shakes, cramps, and tiredness. All these drugs could give you real trouble.

Glue sniffing and other solvent abuse can sometimes lead to chest infections, and liver and kidney damage. People who sniff glue get red marks around the nose and sores around the mouth. The main danger though is of falling off a building or under a car, or drowning, while under the effects of the stuff. Sometimes sniffing butane gas, which is put into lighters, can make you drop down dead.

Using **cocaine** can lead to depression, damage to the inside of your nose, and paranoia. (I had to look that one up. You think everyone hates you. I have that problem all the time, except I don't think it, I know it.)

After all this, had to sit next to the 100-kilo blancmange—Guzzler Guts Gary—at lunch. He's definitely addicted, and not only to food as it turned out. He loosened his tongue and his belt and revealed all, with half the school listening in.

'The first time I had a sniff of glue,' another huge greasy sausage sank between his yellow smelly fangs, 'was with these kids in a multi-storey car park near the local supermarket. I'd already been sniffing gas for a couple of months, so was used to the dizziness, but I kept on blowing on the bag until I blacked out on the floor.' I'm surprised the car park didn't fall down.

'While I was sniffing, I could see all these creatures and ghosts coming out of the walls and things attacking me. When you first sniff glue, there are a few things that can happen. You can fall down dead, be happy or be very depressed. In my case I got depressed. I can't remember why because I was so high on the glue. At the time I really felt like killing myself, then I got used to it and felt good. When I first start-ed, I worried about it a lot. Then it only concerned me when I got ill with stomach pains, or when I started coughing up blood. The only dangerous thing that happened to me was that I was in this park. and was high, and needed some more glue, so I ran across the road to the glue shop and nearly got hit by a bus.' Wonder if the bus knew what a lucky escape it had!

Anyhow Gary has kicked the habit, and thinks there ought to be a law against selling glue to children. I told him he'd gone from glue to grub to greediness to grossness because of his need for 'oral gratification'. Had to explain this meant he liked stuffing his face. He said he could've told me that, so why did I have to use such long words?

Wednesday 15th March
Poured with rain. The 'faded jeans' sex maniacs, alias the drugs police, have disappeared from the school gates, so the girls have stopped hanging around there too.

Friday 17th March
Mum's in a real 'why's everybody getting at me' mood. Been out every night doing her 'good deeds for the neighbourhood' act. Rest of us had a council of war over how to get her to go to bed—one thing she refuses to do when she's wiped out, as

she prefers to drag herself around and be moody with us instead. Dad finally found her asleep in the bath covered with soggy pages of *Women's Own* magazine. She's got awful reading habits but at least she won't need her sleeping tablets tonight.

Next day I couldn't stop myself getting my own back. I told her how Miss 'Big Bum' Court, our sports mistress, didn't think lying in baths was any good for stress and that Mum should be out doing aerobics.

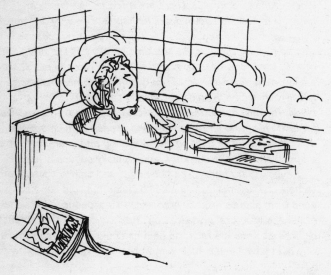

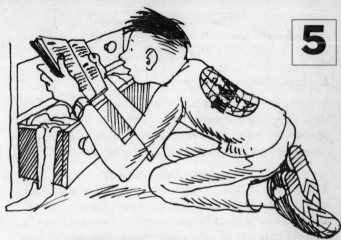

5

Has **Susie** Started **Yet?**

Saturday 18th March

A real find—but I hope nobody reads THIS! Susie's out this morning buying new clothes again with Mum, after moaning about wearing Sally's cast-offs. All she wants these days is to be sorted like her friends. Was desperately looking for my only clean T-shirt, mottoed 'WHY SHOULD I TIDY MY ROOM WHEN THE WORLD'S IN SUCH A MESS?' All my others were dirty and stuffed down the side of my bed as I had as usual forgotten to give them to Mum to wash. Eventually found it in Susie's bottom drawer, PLUS HER DIARY! Didn't mean to read it but it just sort of fell open in my hands.

Tuesday 21st February

Went to Kate's house for the night.

Wednesday 22nd February

Bovril's out all the time. Seems to have a new tom every night. Dad's fed up with the smell they make.

This was really boring. Don't know why girls bother to keep a diary about this sort of thing.

Thursday 23rd February

Kate says she fancies Pete. I told her he picks his nose in the bath.

This was more interesting . . . but Kate. She hardly has tits yet, and anyhow it's not in the bath I pick my nose.

Friday 24th February

Hope Mum and Dad aren't getting divorced. They've had a terrible row. It's all Pete's fault, picking on me as usual. Sally says it's all going to be all right, but I'm not so sure.

Tuesday 28th February

At school today Dave, a real manger who wears shell suits, asked Kate if she'd started yet. She went red and said no and it was none of his business anyway. Later told me she had and that was why she wouldn't go swimming with me last week. Was really miffed that she hadn't told me before.

They started two months ago. She had been staying at her gran's and had had a tummy ache and gone to bed early. In the morning she'd woken up and thought that she'd wet the bed. But it was just a little blood. She'd felt very embarrassed and didn't know what to do with the sheets, but her gran was really nice.

Kate said her mum had told her all about it and she had wanted to start her periods, but now she had, she felt a bit annoyed. Though she was also glad to have joined the other girls who had started in the same year. This definitely made ME feel left out. Anyhow her gran had bought some towels as she didn't have any in the house—her periods had stopped years ago.

Her gran had said that when she was young nobody had told her anything. They called periods the 'curse' and their 'monthlies' and thought they were dirty, and for some reason when they had one weren't even allowed to wash their hair. She had had to wear an awful elastic belt thing to keep a thick towel in place, which felt a bit like wearing a mattress; but luckily she knew that today they have very comfortable, slim 'press on' ones—the very latest style. Kate's mum had also told her all about tampons, and said that it would be perfectly OK to use them, especially if she wanted to go swimming, but Kate wasn't sure she wanted to try them yet.

Kate's lent me a book her mum had got her, called Have You Started Yet? It's good and has lots of people's points of view in it, and tells you in a simple way exactly what happens and how. I think I might get embarrassed discussing periods, but reading about them is fine. I don't know what it'll be like for me. I'm not really scared. I suppose it's just part of growing up. It's funny to think that some of my friends can have babies already. Really strange.

Couldn't find my new pink socks this evening.

Friday 3rd March
Left my homework at school. Watched a really good programme on pets. Wonder if Bovril might have kittens? Still seems to be a kitten herself.

Saturday 4th March
Mum's got no idea. She made me take off all my wet clothes, including my M and S knickers, in the kitchen and run upstairs naked to the bath. I don't think she sees that I might be embarrassed, just because SHE isn't. At least she didn't insist on me sharing a bath with my cousin Daisy, who'd been outside with me and also got soaked.

On the way upstairs Daisy had stared at the lumps on my chest. I'm not really embarrassed by them, but I certainly don't like to be seen with nothing on. My breasts are still very small and hurt a bit when I run. I've got some hair too. Mum's suggested I get a bra, but it's blindingly obvious I've nothing to put in one. I hope they never get as big as Sally's. When she just has a T-shirt on, Pete calls her 'wobbly'. When mine first started to appear I got dead scared. I didn't see myself as that old, but I've got used to it now. Strange to think there's no going back to being a child.

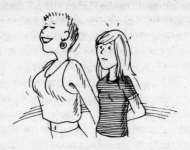

Didn't know that girls get breasts before they start their
periods. My changes seem much less complicated—like my
voice changing. Aunty Pam phoned the other day and started a
long conversation about Uncle Bob's operation, thinking I was
Dad. Anyway, what I said about Sally's tits is true.

Sunday 5th March

*Have read some more of Have You Started Yet? Pete always
seemed to be around just when I was going to talk to Mum
about it. But Mum got the message, and when we went to
visit Uncle Bob in hospital, she suggested that Pete should
stay behind and catch up with his homework.*

*As we were driving there, I asked when I was likely to start
my periods as my breasts were getting bigger since
Christmas. The book said that most girls begin between the
ages of 9 and 17. Mum told me that some girls get their
periods almost as soon as their breasts appear, and some
only after several years, but both are normal. She told me that
at first I shouldn't expect my periods to happen every month. I
might have just a few spots of blood and then nothing for a
bit. When they settled down the amount of blood I would lose
would be about a third of a mugful each time. Although most
women get periods every month, a few women get them every
three weeks, and a few every six weeks. Also, the time a period
lasts varies between one or two days and a week. Mum said
she'd get me a packet of sanitary towels just to be prepared.*

At the hospital we gave Uncle Bob the flowers we had got. The place smelt awful, like an overclean public lavatory, and Uncle Bob was really embarrassing. 'I bet you have all the boys chasing after you, you're becoming a real woman now, aren't you?' I wasn't going to tell HIM I haven't started yet!

Monday 6th March

Some more time for reading this evening. Funny to think there are two hundred thousand little eggs sitting around in my ovaries. Even though over my whole lifetime, only 400 or so will ever get released. Seems an awful waste. Every month, hormone messages from my brain will tell my ovaries to release an egg. If the egg doesn't meet a sperm and get fertilized (help, that's not going to happen to mine for a long time yet) then whoosh, out of my vagina it comes, along with the cells and blood from the lining of my uterus. It sounds rather like flushing the loo.

Kate says she wishes there was a button you could press and it would all come out at once, instead of messily dribbling out over several days. She thinks tampons and sanitary towels should be free on the National Health Service. What's also clever is the way the brain sends different hormone messages when you get pregnant, so that you don't have a period and the lining of your uterus stays all spongy and ready for the fertilized egg to start growing there into a baby.

Tuesday 7th March

Had a stomach ache today. Kept rushing to the loo to see if I'd started, especially as I felt a bit wet down there. It was nothing except a bit of what the book calls 'normal vaginal discharge'. Sometimes this happens before you have a period, so it might be going to happen to me soon. Hope so. My only worry now is WHERE I start. Hope it doesn't happen when I go swimming.

Am fed up with all the old clothes I have to wear. They make me look totally shapeless.

Wednesday 8th March

The stomach ache turned out to be the diarrhoea squits. Must have caught it from Jane, who was off school with the same thing. Pete's his usual awful self. 'Ugh! Don't come near me with your dirty germs. Hope you've washed your hands after the loo. That's how these things get spread, you know.' As if I didn't know. Mum was nice though. Told me not to eat and just have lots of small drinks of water and coke until my guts have recovered and can cope with food again. Now I'm starving.

Missed all the drama at school about drugs.

Thursday 9th March

Mum's very touchy. Perhaps she's got PMT like I read about in the book. Pete thought PMT stood for Pre-Menstrual Tantrums. Could see what he meant, but he's such a 'know all', I didn't put him right.

I'm sure it means Pre-Menstrual Tantrums. It must be Susie who has it wrong. I'll have to look it up. Anyhow, I bet it was just Mum having a bit of diarrhoea.

Friday 10th March

Not PMT (perhaps I will tell Pete that it stands for pre-menstrual tension), just the squits like me. Heard Mum going to the loo all night. Hope she's better tomorrow so we can go shopping.

Saturday 11th March

Only got lovely new red and blue swimsuit from Top Shop as Mum's a bit short of money this week and didn't have the energy to traipse round many shops. Hate those communal changing rooms. Seemed like everyone was looking at me. Tried it on without taking my shirt off, and with Mum telling me not to be silly, we're all the same. We jolly well aren't. For instance, Liz has tiny breasts and huge nipples. Her new bikini emphasizes her Egyptian look. The boys all call her 'pyramid', and say things like she would have to sleep on her back on a water bed or she'd puncture it. She's very tall and wishes her pituitary gland would concentrate on making her grow outwards rather than upwards. Still, according to Kate, she spent all her time hanging about the school gates when the drug policemen were there, so her hormones must be doing something.

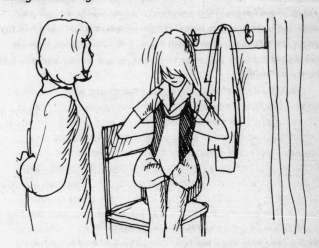

Sunday 12th March

Uncle Bob's out of hospital and Mum and Dad have gone off to visit. Couldn't face any more of his embarrassing remarks myself. Wandered into Sally's room to try on one of her bras, but she was there. She started to tease me about not starting yet.

She said that before she started she was jealous of all her friends who had. Her best friend had taken her into a corner and told her about it, like it was some incredible secret and terribly exciting. Another of her friends had really bad period pains, and if Sally was nasty to her at all she looked at her pityingly and said, 'Look, when you're a woman you'll understand the pain and anguish it causes.' Sally said,

'A woman! She was only 13.'

When Sally had started it was a Tuesday, suitably enough just after biology, and she was a bit alarmed but also excited. She was too embarrassed to tell any of her friends, because when she thought about it, it seemed a pretty foul idea. It didn't cause her much trouble at first, no tummy pains or pre-menstrual tension or anything, but later she started getting occasional tummy cramps with her periods and took paracetamol, which helped. Now the doctor gives her some tablets, because the cramps are worse and she has this swollen feeling.

Sally told me about how to use tampons, which was just as well because I couldn't see how I would ever get them in. She said she had found them difficult, and hadn't put them far enough up because she thought they would get lost inside. Then she'd discovered that there are two kinds of tampon. Some have applicators—shiny white cardboard tubes around them. These slip in easily. You then pull out the cardboard, leaving the tampon in the right place in your vagina. The others are without applicators. You just have to push them in until they feel comfortable. Both kinds come with a diagram showing how to use them. And both have a thread attached to the bottom of the tampon, to pull it out with.

I was just finishing when the front door slammed and Mum shouted 'Pete' up the stairs, so I stuffed the diary back, blushing like mad. Back to picking my nose in the bog.

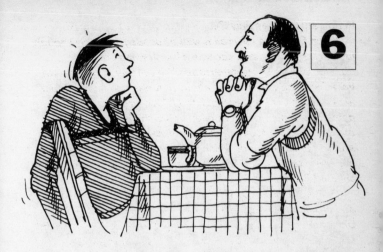

6

My own **'Life Changes'**, but They Take a Long Time

Sunday 19th March

Have to be careful what I say in front of Susie or she'll wonder how I know, but I'm glad I don't have periods. Wish that my voice breaking just happened like that though, overnight. For months now when I open my mouth I'm not sure what's going to come out, a foghorn or a squeak.

My changes must be obvious to everyone because Dad keeps trying to bring up the subject of puberty and 'the facts of life'. Must have been him that left the book about sex and puberty in my room. This morning he started to tell me about what he called 'the birds and the bees', so I informed him I knew it all already—to help him out, as I began to feel as embarrassed as he seemed. He looked relieved and rushed off to the garage. I really feel for Dad sometimes. I wonder if Mum's behind all this concern? I'd have thought she had enough to worry about with Susie's changes. Don't know why grown-ups want to talk about those things all the time. Think Mum and Dad must be obsessed with sex.

Monday 20th March

Had to go with Dad to see Uncle Bob this evening. He seems to be surviving OK. Managed not to let on I knew why Susie and Mum didn't want me to go last time. All that women's talk, but I'm afraid Dad is cornering me for the same reason. Uncle Bob seems to have a one-track mind too. His first words were, 'Got yourself a girlfriend yet?', and he promised me a razor for my next birthday. I'd rather have the money. But what even Dad embarrassingly refers to as 'your moustache' is definitely going to need a scrape soon. The hairs under my arms, and around my willy, haven't been slow in growing either, but I don't worry about them—I just wear long shirts. Problem is that I'm still very short.

I haven't talked to anyone about it all, except jokingly with my friends. It gets a bit mean sometimes, like James saying that Randy Jo thought he'd grown a pubic hair till he discovered it was his prick. Suppose we're all going through it together. Mostly we choose to ignore it, as we're too embarrassed to talk

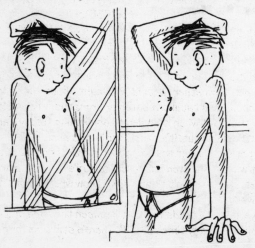

about it. Somehow, being 'inside' myself makes me feel completely different about my own changes than about my friends' changes.

Thursday 30th March

Feeling bored. Tried to find Susie's diary again. It's not there. Has she guessed? Knowing her, she's probably dusted it for fingerprints.

Friday 7th April

Discovered! After school Susie disappeared. At supper she gave us all meaningful looks and announced she'd bought a diary with a lock on. Mum suggested she could look after the spare key if Susie wanted, and then suddenly went bright red.

Tuesday 11th April

Have taken to hiding MY diary under my mattress.

Tuesday 18th April

Spent Easter with Sam's family in Wales. Forgot to take my diary as it was under my mattress.

Monday 24th April

Back to school. Whole world suddenly sex obsessed, though at school it's called 'Life Changes' or 'PSE' or 'Human Reproduction'. Had a 'Now no sniggering while I put this on the blackboard' class today, all about the physical facts.

Dad had to sign a letter saying it was OK for them to teach me about sex at school. I told Dad I didn't think it was right for him to decide whether I should be taught about sex or not. I can do without being taught geography, or maths—he's welcome to decide that. But when it comes to something I really want (and need) to know about, it's stupid for him to decide.

I'm not sure I want to know about it from Mr Rogers though. I doubt whether he even has a sex life. Raj's parents didn't sign their letter—so I don't think Raj will know where to put it when he grows up.

Boys' puberty tends to start between the ages of 10 and 13, and finishes at any time up to 18. There's still time for me then, as I'm shorter than many of my friends. Even the girls are taller, but apparently on average they start their changes two years ahead of us boys.

In boys, the first thing is our balls get bigger, and over three years they increase seven times in size. Next comes pubic hair, and bits of hair under our arms, and with some of us hair on our chests too. Hope I don't get hair on my chest. Nothing much I can do about it if I do. Wonder if anyone shaves there? Then our height goes shooting up—can't be too soon for me. We grow a quarter of our final height during this time. Finally our penis grows in length. All these things start at different times in different boys, go on for different lengths of time, and occur in different orders. In one way, we all end up the same after we've been through puberty, but in another we all end up different, because we still have different sizes and shapes and looks.

Lots of other changes are going on too. Our muscles are getting bigger and heavier, our shoulders broader, our voices deeper. This is something to do with bigger vocal cords. Like Susie's changes, all these things in boys are controlled by chemicals called hormones produced in the brain.

The diagrams and description of male parts and an erection on the board made it all look unreal, in fact a bit like a pneumatic pump. It seems there are muscles which stop the blood flowing out of the penis, but go on letting the blood flow in. More and more blood fills it up, making it bigger and longer—a bit like an elongated balloon.

We were also taught how vulnerable and short the life of a poor sperm is. Sperms die very easily if they get too hot or too cold. No wonder our testes have to increase seven times— about 100,000,000 sperms in 3 millilitres of fluid come out each time we make love or masturbate (just under a teaspoonful), though only one is needed to fertilize an egg. Seems a fantastic waste. It's funny how difficult it is to connect all this with my own body. Mr Rogers, of 'PSE' fame, said this was only the physical side of things, and a talk about 'feelings', about sex and love, would take place on Friday.

Tuesday 25th April

If we have greasy chips and hamburgers one more time for
school lunch I'll go mad (or get Mum to make me packed
lunches). The sex obsession goes on. I scored by bringing in
Dad's book. Everyone pretended not to be interested but they
all looked at the bit on 'Normal Size of Penises'. It said:

The majority of boys and men think that their penis is too small and
it is very difficult sometimes to convince them otherwise. So an
American doctor has done some research, using a ruler to measure
the length of the non-erect penis of boys and men of different ages.

AGE	RANGE OF PENILE LENGTH
10	4 to 8 cms
12	5 to 10 cms
14	6 to 14 cms
16	10 to 15 cms
18	11 to 17 cms

For most men and boys it was found that however small the non-
erect penis was, penises were all roughly the same length when
erect.

Mine goes straight from a floppy start of 11.2 cms to a
standing finish of 15.4 cms in 30 seconds . . . It obviously
hasn't reached its maximum acceleration or length yet. I
wonder what I'd get an Olympic gold medal for?

Wednesday 26th April

Slight sore throat, so tried to look as ill as possible and told
Mum about it. Usual sympathy from her, which means taking
my temperature, finding it normal, giving me two paracetamol
and ordering me to school. Threw up all over the floor in class
and got sent home. Hope this made Mum feel really guilty.

Thursday 27th April

Now Mum's convinced I am DESPERATELY ill. Still wouldn't call
the doctor though. Said it was probably just a viral infection
and I'd soon be better. Sam said it must be meningitis as I had

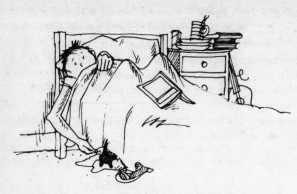

a headache. Had to spend boring day in bed. Felt fine by the evening but not allowed to go out. Don't think it can be meningitis, but I think I'm getting pimples on my nose. Bovril's had her kittens in the dirty clothes under my bed. Susie's furious because she missed seeing them come out.

Friday 28th April

Back to school, and it turned out the talk on 'Feelings' was to be just a film called *Personal Relationships*. Typical grown-ups' views on what they think we're thinking. Managed to get some of it right though. It tried to say that at our age we tend to:

* lose interest in things that our parents organize for us, and are more reluctant to accept advice and criticism (just like Susie, in fact).
* feel concerned about, but also uncertain about, our appearance and whether we are attractive in other people's eyes (this applies to me).
* have times when we feel totally bored, unwanted by everyone, and have nothing to do, when everyone else seems to be having a really good time (too right).
* feel good about the world one day and totally upset by it the next.
* worry about whether we are ever going to get to know a girlfriend or boyfriend really well (like Cilla and me).

* think we are different from everyone else, but at the same time desperately want to be the same.
* worry whether our sexual feelings are normal. (Are they too strong or too weak, should we be worrying about masturbation and wet dreams, the size of our penises, our breasts, and when our periods are going to start?)

In the discussion afterwards I said I didn't think that we WERE all that interested in ourselves, and it seemed it was the grown-ups who were more interested than us. It was obvious from the questions that some of my friends didn't even know what wet dreams are.

Mr Rogers said that there is a lot of variation in interest in sex, and whether you feel attracted to people of the opposite sex or the same sex, and that some people think about it a lot and others not at all, and all are normal. Then he explained that wet dreams are sexy dreams during which you ejaculate or 'come' while still asleep. They are called 'wet' dreams because you wet the bed with your sperm. He went on to explain that many boys and girls find that masturbation is 'a harmless and very pleasant way of relieving feelings of sexual tension' and that you aren't over-sexed if you do masturbate, wank, pull yourself off, beat your salami, toss off, or whatever else you call it, and aren't undersexed if you don't.

What was good was that Mr Rogers was not at all embarrassed when talking about these things. Amazing to think that EVERY person that one EVER sees is the result of two people making love and a sperm fertilizing an egg—even Mr Rogers! Looked at everyone in school with new eyes. I wonder if Mum and Dad still do it—grim.

Tuesday 2nd May

Caught out by Mum again. After my bicycle accident she bought me these really gross black leather school shoes to wear, instead of my ruined white trainers. I'd been outsmarting her by changing into the trainers in the garage on the way to school. Got back today to change into Mum's shoes and found them with a note saying, 'Wear them or there's no pocket money,' signed 'Your Mother'. Luckily I know she'll forget, and with luck I'll be able to wear my old trainers and have my pocket money as well. She's really safe sometimes.

Friday 5th May
Was right—Mum's forgotten. Cycled to school in my trainers. Decided to ask Cilla if she'd come to the cinema on Sunday.

Saturday 6th May
Cilla's already going with Randy Jo. Feel a complete failure.

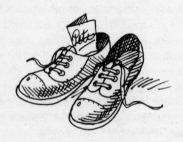

7

Learning to **Live** with my **Zits**

Tuesday 9th May

Weekend got worse and worse. Pimples have turned into real
spots. Every time I looked another had appeared. My skin's
gone all greasy, with lumps around my nose. It's disgusting.
Dad's sympathetic, but he's not much help. Said, 'Oh, it's just
acne. Everyone gets it when they're young.' JUST! That isn't
much help to someone with a face covered in molehills. He went
on about how they would clear up soon, but they haven't gone
yet. Actually they're worse. Tried squeezing them and although I
got something out, it's made them flare up. Some seem to have
black heads, others have white heads. Maybe I don't wash
enough.

Wednesday 10th May

A black day in my life at school. Cilla said, 'Ugh, what have you
done to your face?' I thought that would have been obvious. She
wears so much make-up, you'd need a spade to find out what
was going on on her skin. Called her 'Pancake Face', which hardly
improved our relationship. Not that it was much good anyway.

Thursday 11th May

They're spreading. Slogs was kind enough to point it out to me after games today. Said my back looked like a pizza. Checked in the mirror. He's right. Where are they going to spread to next?

Friday 12th May

Good old Mum. Thought she hadn't noticed. She left a tube of cream in my room after tea, plus an article she'd found in an old Sunday colour supplement. It's called 'A Spot of Bother' and seems to know what it's talking about.

'Acne happens most commonly in young people because of the surge in hormones that comes with puberty. It tends to be worse in boys (just my luck) and affects the face and shoulders most, because that's where hair follicles are commonest.

There are a lot of myths about what causes acne. It isn't caused by eating too much sugar or chips; nor by masturbation (I'm relieved about that, as I had begun to think that was why me and most of my friends had zits). Nor do people get acne because they don't wash enough. Washing your face twice a day with soap and water should help in most cases, especially if you use a medicated soap that contains an antiseptic. However these soaps will help only mild cases, and you need to use them for several weeks.

Some shampoos, foundation creams, moisturizers and hair conditioners can make acne worse—particularly those which are heavy and greasy. (I'll pass some of this on to Cilla.) Eye make-up, lipstick, powders, blushers, and toilet waters, on the other hand, shouldn't cause you any problems.

One thing that you can try for yourself to help your acne is to go out in the sun. Sunlight is usually good for spots. It reduces the number of bacteria in the skin, encourages peeling (Ugh) to get rid of the horny layer of skin, loosens blackheads, and decreases the rate at which sebum is produced . . .'

Still don't really understand why I have got them, or what 'sebum' is, but it doesn't sound at all nice.

Saturday 13th May

Aunty Pam's coming tomorrow! Horror. Maybe she won't kiss me now I've got acne. That's the only advantage I can think of. Put

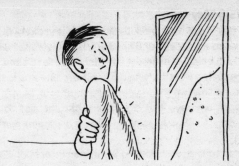

the cream on for the second time today. Amazed there's no improvement.

Mum and Dad went out for an hour, leaving me to 'baby-sit' for Susie, a term she doesn't exactly like. Told her it was exactly right though, as she still spends a lot of time making clothes for her Sindy doll. She'll begin to look like one of them soon. Tried persuading Mum and Dad to pay me. They refused with an argument about how they didn't make me pay for my meals, so offered to go and eat at MacDonalds.

Sunday 14th May

Aunty Pam came and gave me the kiss of Dracula, despite the fact that I'm covered in zits. Hope they ARE catching. Wonder where I can find out more about acne? Might try the library's dictionary again. Is there a magic cure?

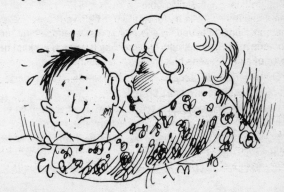

Monday 15th May

Dictionary not much help. Said it was a *'skin eruption with red pimples'*. Makes my face sound like a volcano. In despair about the cream I am using. It seems a complete waste of time, but the article said it's worth trying different creams and lotions till you find one that works on your particular skin. Mum's got me this new lotion. Says it's cheaper, and the chemist told her there is nothing to show that more expensive creams work better.

Rushed up to the bathroom to try it, as the school disco is in two weeks' time and I'm getting desperate. Embarrassing enough to ask a girl to dance, let alone if you've got acne. The lotion stung a bit when I put it on, so I looked at the instructions to make sure I was doing it right. There was a long leaflet giving all the facts.

Apparently 70 per cent of the teenage population have acne at one time or another. It's not a disease but just a normal part of growing up.

It usually disappears between the ages of 16 and 25. You can get acne anywhere you have hairs (ANYWHERE? I hope not) because it is in the hair follicles that it starts, but it mainly affects the face, back, shoulders and chest (what a relief).

It isn't catching—so much for my revenge on Aunty Pam— and my fantasies about kissing a girl can continue.

'Sebum' is a substance secreted by the sebaceous glands, next to the hair follicles. Apparently a normal amount of sebum helps keep the skin slightly oily and protects it from wetness, bacteria and other things, but too much gives the skin the greasiness I find so gross.

Some girls have acne worse at the times of their periods. (At least I don't have that trouble.)

It's easier to use an electric razor with acne than to shave with soap. (Will Dad let me use his when I need one?)

Washing with an antiseptic soap helps. (Must get Mum to get me some of that as well.)

It's better not to squeeze spots because they tend to get

infected and you may end up with more. But if you do have to fiddle with them (and who doesn't?) make sure your hands are clean and only squeeze the blackheads. It even explained why blackheads are black. Apparently it's nothing to do with dirt— just a bit of pigment from the skin.

At the end it said, 'Most mild acne clears either without treatment or after using a cream or lotion. If it doesn't, it is advisable to consult your family doctor, who can prescribe other forms of treatment.'

While reading all this, kept looking in the mirror to see if the lotion was working. Then noticed leaflet said that it might take several days. Went to bed.

Friday 26th May
Even Susie has noticed my zits are a bit better. Just as well, as it's the school disco tonight. I've nearly forgotten what I look like without spots. I don't think my friends would recognize me if they all disappeared. Anyway I'll keep on with the soap even if they do. Noticed today that even Randy Jo has a few zits. Doesn't seem to have put the girls off though. Maybe because most of them have spots too.

Went to the disco. It turned out to be too dark to have to worry about how we looked. Danced once with Cilla but didn't get anywhere.

Sally's **Sex Life** Goes Wrong

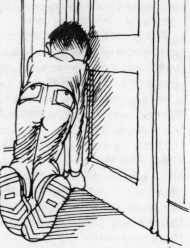

Saturday 27th May

Couldn't sleep last night—a tad hot about Cilla—though I was really tired. Often can't sleep these days. It's incredibly annoying and seems to come in runs of a few nights at a time. I worry that I'm not getting all the sleep I need, and am going to be tired and grumpy and no good at anything next day. I've tried relaxing and counting sheep jumping over fences and reading my old books (new books, like Cilla, make me too excited because I want to know what's going to happen next). I think that I'm never going to get to sleep and so I don't.

Mum says that I don't get enough exercise. I've read somewhere that having sex is the equivalent exercise of running a mile, but I doubt if my own efforts on myself demand the same energy.

Finally thought I'd go and get a hot drink. It was midnight and everyone should've been in bed. Was about to go into the kitchen when I heard Mum and Sally behind the door. Sally was crying and saying she thought she might be pregnant. I couldn't believe my ears. Someone has scored with my sister! My ear found itself glued to the door and wouldn't come away.

MUM: Here, have a hanky. For God's sake, haven't you been using something, after all we talked about?
SAL: I didn't think anything was going to happen, did I? We were at a party and had been drinking. It only happened once, and I wasn't going to take the Pill all these months, on the chance it might happen sometime, was I? Anyway, if I had been taking it, Mike might have thought I was an easy pull.
MUM: Why didn't you ask him to use something then? It was just as much his responsibility as yours.
SAL: Couldn't stop half-way through and ask him.
MUM: You bloody well could have and should have. Or you should have got emergency contraception. You could have gone to any doctor and you can use it up to 72 hours afterwards. However, it's a bit late now.
SAL: What are we going to do? Please, please don't tell Dad. I feel so stupid.
MUM: Best thing is for us to go to the doctor on Monday, and then we'll . . .

I gave up my hot drink at this point and retired upstairs. I can see why they're discussing putting condom machines in the sixth-form toilets at school. I was now more insomniac than ever, but insomnia was a minor problem compared with Sal's.

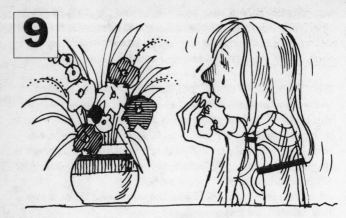

Susie Gets **Hayfever**

Monday 29th May

Susie's revolting. Her sniffing sounds like a pig with indigestion. Said I'd have my breakfast in the other room because I couldn't stand it any longer. So Susie screamed and burst into tears, while Mum made a face at me for being unsympathetic. Nobody was amused when I said it was like sitting next to a vacuum cleaner gone wrong. Couldn't stop thinking about all that yukky green snot being sucked down the back of her throat.

Wednesday 31st May

Susie's still sniffing. Hope I don't catch her cold. Bovril's no longer feeding her kittens, and is off playing with the toms again. Sally's not having a baby and has bust up with Mike. It's official (via the kitchen door).

Thursday 1st June

Now it's Susie's sneezing, snoring and sniffling all night that's stopping me getting to sleep. No toilet paper in the loo and it's obvious why. Susie's room and the rest of the house are covered with a snow of crumpled white tissues. It's better than her sniffing anyway. Sally says she bets it's not a cold, but hayfever, like she gets herself sometimes. Whatever it is, I still hope I don't catch it.

Saturday 3rd June

A lovely sunny day. Reluctantly persuaded on to a tennis court by Sam, who said it would be good for my health. Susie's flopping around the house looking red-eyed, as if she's been crying all night, and says she's got a terrible headache. Beaten by Sam of course.

Had my weekly bath (under threat of no pocket money from Mum) listening to the radio. There was this 'phone in' on hayfever. Sally was right, this is what Susie has. There's a lot of it around at the moment, on account of the 'pollen count' being high because of the weather. This pollen is made up of seeds that come from trees and grasses during the spring and summer, especially on a hot sunny day after rainy weather. The runny nose, sneezing and itchy eyes are the body's way of trying to get rid of this pollen stuff.

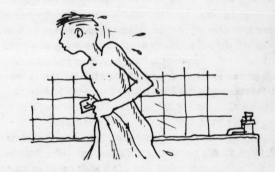

Got me wondering why all this wasn't happening to me, so I leapt out of the bath leaving a trail of wet footprints, with a towel round my privates to make me half-decent (I wasn't having anyone seeing ME, even if half the rest of my family like going around exposing themselves). I marched downstairs to the phone, my stomach in my mouth from nerves. But I had to find out, and suddenly there I was on the radio, hoping that at least one of my friends was listening to my radio début so that they could broadcast the fact in school on Monday.

'Is,' I wanted to know, 'hayfever catching, and how come I don't have it?' Madam Clever Doc on the other end of the line put on her most tolerant medical voice: *'What a good question. How old are you and may we know your name?'* '18 and my name's Sam', I lied, suddenly losing my nerve. Explosive laughter from Susie who had appeared from nowhere between sneezes.

'Well, Sam, hayfever is a kind of allergy, which means that your body becomes very sensitive to certain substances. These substances, like pollens, are called allergens and when they get into your body, some of the white cells in your blood produce complicated chemical substances called antibodies to get rid of them. When the allergens and antibodies meet they produce a reaction which brings about the release of a substance called histamine, and it's this that causes hayfever sufferers to sneeze and have runny eyes. Nobody knows why some people have this special sensitivity to things like pollens. And I thought it was me that was meant to be sensitive. *Usually antibodies are good things to have, as they help fight off bacteria which cause many diseases.'*

'About one in ten people have hayfever, and although it tends to run in families, you don't catch it from someone else. Some people are born with a tendency to have it.' Couldn't waste the chance, so asked her how I could stop my sister's nose from running. Could she use corks?

Susie hacked my ankle while the voice down the phone said, *'Well, Sam, that's another good question.'* (Mrs Smellie could learn something from her.) *'There is a wide range of things that you can do, though corking your nose isn't one of them. There are also medicines that you can take. It's very unfortunate that exams are often held at the same time of year as the hayfever season. If your sister's taking exams, she should go and see your own family doctor and get some treatment. If it's really bad, the doctor may even give her a note for the teacher.'* She added that this couldn't be used as an excuse for getting poor marks unless the hayfever was very bad. I decided that I wanted to hear MY voice again.

'But what about my sister's nose? That's the real problem.' **'Well, if antihistamines don't help,'** she said, **'there are special sprays on prescription from your doctor, which your sister can squirt up her nose.'** Was just going to ask about some of Susie's other nasty habits when the radio presenter said, **'Well, thank you very much Sam, and our next question comes from a Mrs Snodgrass.'**

She deserved to have hayfever with a name like that. Her question was about other kinds of treatment than those given by doctors. Apparently all sorts of things have been tried for hayfever. You can try hypnotism, acupuncture, homeopathy and other things. At the end of the programme they said to write for a special pack explaining all about hayfever. Told Susie that I'd do that for her. She looked very surprised—it's not often that I am so helpful to my sister.

Sunday 4th June

Went to the Heath for a picnic, along with five million others who haven't anything better to do with their Sundays. Watched some grown-ups playing at being children with radio-controlled,

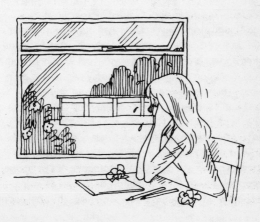

perfect-scale, 'better than the real thing' model boats. Posers. What could have been a great picnic was ruined by Susie feeling miserable.

On the way back all agreed that it must be hayfever, and that Mum should take Susie to the doctor's first thing on Monday morning. Got away with watching telly half the evening as everyone was fussing over Susie.

To take Susie's mind off her nose, I told her how in our PSE class Mr Rogers had told us about the biggest study of sex that had ever happened in Britain. She asked whether I'd been part of it, so I said my questionnaire had got lost in the post. I didn't tell her it would've been blank anyhow! I wasn't sure Mum would approve, but *I* thought Susie should have the facts.

The study showed that although most people seem to think that 16-year-olds are all at it, in fact by the age of 15 only about 3 in every 100 girls and 9 in every 100 boys had had sex; and by the age of 16 only 18 in every 100 girls and 27 in every 100 boys had done it. This was a bit of relief for me because hearing people talk, I think me and half my class expected to have bonked by now! It seems we're just normal.

Mr Rogers also said that most people seemed to have their first sexual experience—snogging, cuddling, petting—around 13 years of age. (In my case, it wasn't for not trying with Cilla, but I didn't like to ask about Susie's experiences.)

One thing I didn't think Susie was old enough for was what he told us about homosexuality—boys or men fancying one another and girls or women fancying one another. That doesn't seem all that common either, with only about 6 in every 100 men and 3 in every 100 women having had any kind of homosexual experience. This certainly took away some of my worries, because every time one of the sixth-form boys looked at me I was beginning to feel a bit nervous. Mr Rogers said that if you were in a boys-only, or girls-only, school, the sex drive was so strong that if you didn't have someone of the opposite sex to experiment with, then it might easily lead to doing something with someone of your own sex—but only about 1 in every 100 men and 1 in every 200 women are homosexual as adults.

Monday 5th June

It's half-term, and Sally has been in charge while Mum and Dad are out working. It's not fair, when Sally 'baby-sits', she gets paid.

Instead of being her usual bossy self, Sally was actually quite nice. Turned out that she used to suffer from hayfever quite badly. The attacks got bad again last year, when she started riding on the back of Mike's motorbike, and going out into the fields. She ignored me when I asked what they did in the fields.

To keep my end up, and not feel left out of all this hayfever 'know how', I started to tell Sally about the radio programme. She wasn't interested till I told her it was just as well she hadn't got her own motorbike yet, because if you sneeze at 60 miles an hour, your eyes can be closed for half a second, during which you travel 44 feet blind.

Tuesday 6th June

Feel sorry for Susie. She's being teased at school. Her teacher said she was just putting it on, and didn't listen when she asked to be moved away from an open window to get away from the pollen. A friend had called her 'cry baby' when she saw her red eyes. Susie explained that it was just hayfever, but her friend said, 'That's what they all say.' Finally, she had come fourth in the 400 metres race, all because she had felt so awful, with a streaming nose and watering eyes. This was something she was normally CHAMPION at.

It makes me feel really angry for Susie, people teasing her. I also hate anyone bullying anyone else. It seems to me there's enough meanness in the world, like Bosnia and all that, without making it happen in school.

Friday 9th June

Loo paper's back where it should be and the sniffing rate has dropped drastically. Susie's a different person—back to her usual argumentative self. Think I'M becoming allergic to my sisters. They're determined to reduce me to having streaming eyes too. Am going back to worrying about the more important things in life—like my zits, and how to get up courage to ask Cilla out.

Saturday 10th June

Thought I'd found a friend at last! A lovely thick envelope with my name on it arrived today—definitely not the usual reminder from the library about overdue books. Opened it with great expectations and found it was just stuff for Susie on hayfever.

Hayfever: The facts

(1) There are 6,000,000 people who suffer from hayfever in England.
(2) There is no cure, though medicines help to prevent and treat it, and some people do grow out of it. This may not happen till you are 30 or 40.

This seems really ancient to me.

(3) There are skin tests where they inject you with a small extract of the pollens (in other allergies they use other substances like house dust, or animal fur) usually on your arm. Some minutes later, if you are allergic, you get a small itchy swelling in the place where the prick is made. However, skin tests don't always work and they sometimes show that you seem to be allergic to a lot more things than you actually are.

What can be done to make it less uncomfortable?

The best way not to get hayfever is to avoid pollen; but this may not always be possible and in many cases it is better to treat it than become a hermit. Ten handy tips which help are:

✓ Stay away from grassy areas.
✓ Take your holidays by the sea.
✓ Keep your house windows closed when your neighbours mow the grass.
✓ Remember there is more pollen about on hot days.
✓ Wear dark glasses out of doors.
✓ Avoid taking walks in the evening.

✓ Avoid trips in the countryside in June and July.
✓ Keep the car windows closed when driving.
✓ Check the pollen forecast.
✓ Ask your doctor for advice and be sure to take the medicine prescribed. Antihistamines are the most common ones, but they can make you feel a bit sleepy.

Might use this information to earn some extra pocket money by offering my services to the local radio station.

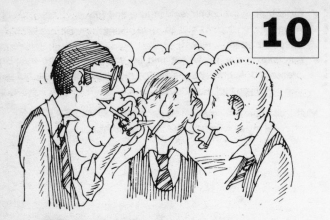

My **First Fag** Nearly Kills Me

Wednesday 14th June

Feeling hard done by the last few days. My mates have all gone on a school field trip to Cornwall. Only twenty places and I wasn't given one of them. We're having to WORK while they're having a good time, and we're being taught by really wet teachers while all the good ones are off enjoying themselves on the trip. There's nothing on telly except Neighbours, and all the films are PG and not worth seeing.

After school, didn't particularly want to go home as Susie had gone to stay with Kate again, and Mum and Dad were going to be away till late on Dad's department's outing. Hope it will make them be nicer to one another, as they've been having more of their so-called 'discussions' recently.

I was unwillingly drifting home, with nothing much to do, when I saw what appeared to be smoke signals going up from the Rec. I couldn't read the signals so went to investigate (this was me in my private detective role). It turned out to be some of my classmates trying to kill themselves with fags. Before I could open my mouth, they shouted, 'Here comes "know all" Pete' and ' "I know what's good for you" Pete' and ' "You're killing yourselves" Pete'. They cornered me, puffing smoke in my face and chanting, 'Yeh—we know, we know—don't cack yer pants, Pete.'

It seems utterly stupid to me that they still smoke, when they know full well:

* It kills you—actively, and all those around you—passively
* By the time we grow up, smoking will kill 10 million of us around the world each year
* If we have four friends who smoke, at least two will die from it
* In the UK, smoking kills nearly as many as a load of passengers on a Boeing 747, EVERY DAY
* Every cigarette knocks five minutes off our lives
* It damages babies inside the womb
* Kissing a smoker is like kissing an ashtray.

What a load of tossers.

They were perfectly happy to yabber on about WHY they smoked. Ann said that she started when she was 13. Her older sister was going out with a heavy smoker. One night her boyfriend visited their house when their parents were out and he and her sister went to the back door (their mum wouldn't allow the smell inside the house) and began to smoke. EastEnders had finished so she went outside too. Her sister said jokingly, 'Would you like a cigarette?' and she said OK, because she didn't want to look stupid in front of the boyfriend. Smoking was very strange and made her feel dizzy and hurt the back of her throat, but she carried on to impress her sister and the boyfriend. Now she got her fags from the corner shop, or bummed them off her friends.

Dave said that he got his fags from lots of different shops and though he was only 14, he never had any trouble buying them.

He enjoyed smoking and thought it made him look big and hard, and said that if someone wanted to smoke it was up to them and nothing to do with anyone else. He started smoking when he and his cousin bought some cigarettes and tried them down by the river. He didn't like them much and at first only smoked at parties and discos. Later he had a lot of arguments with his mother and used to get very upset, but found that a fag 'sort of helped'. He hated girls smoking, as he thought it made them look common. Once at school he nearly got caught so he stuffed the fag into his pocket and burnt himself. Silly bastard.

Ann butted in here and said she didn't see why girls smoking was any different from boys. She thought it made HER look big and hard, and it kept her thin and made her sexier, which mattered more than dying a bit sooner. This is stupid of her. I know loads of thin people who don't smoke and anyhow, according to Sam's dad, it's not so much the dying early that matters, but the falling to pieces, bit by bit, all the time that you're smoking. She didn't think there was any point in her giving up, as her mum and dad smoked and her health was still in danger because she was breathing in their smoke. She didn't seem to care what happened in twenty years' time, as we'd probably all be dead from toxic waste.

Some kid that I had never talked to before said that he smoked at school every day and never got caught. He and his friends kept their lighted cigarettes in their desks and lifted up the top when they wanted a drag. He didn't think that the teachers cared much, as most of them smoked, and you could smell Mr Rogers's smoky breath from half a mile away. This kid wished he didn't smoke because it was crippling him financially— but he couldn't stop, especially as all his friends did it.

In the end they insisted on me having one, so that I knew what I was missing. They suggested that there was something wrong with me if I didn't smoke—or was it that I was too soft to try? Although I actually thought it would be bigger and harder of me NOT to try, I didn't risk saying so and had a drag, which didn't feel too bad, though it made me want to cough. In my role as detective, I took two or three more really deep ones—and the top of my head began to fall off. I started coughing and getting pins and needles feelings in my hands. My eyes watered and I nearly fainted away. When I began to look as if I was about to throw up, my classmates, who had been killing themselves laughing, edged away.

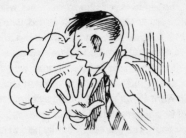

On the way home a ditty kept going through my mind, over and over again. 'The smoker is a silly tit, the fags just make you stink like shit.' I stopped at the local shop to buy five packets of polos and some chewing gum to cover up the smell. All I could see were packets and packets of cigarettes and endless adverts. And when I came out, staring me in the face across the road was a picture, twenty feet high, of a bit of purple silk with a slit in it, advertising some fags called 'Silk Cut'. In TINY letters at the bottom it said 'DANGER—SMOKING CAN KILL'. It was only twenty-five yards from the local primary school entrance. Really sad—having it so close, where little kids can see it.

What a lot of arseholes. Why does the government let cigarette companies have adverts, if smoking damages you?

Got home, cleaned my teeth, ate a packet of polos, and held my breath when Mum kissed me goodnight.

Thursday 15th June
Came top in the maths test. Had a Mars Bar to celebrate. Worried about a pain in my groin. Think it must be appendicitis but according to the medical dictionary I should have a temperature and be throwing up, so it can't be that.

Saturday 17th June

Spent morning reading Sam's old bicycle magazines. He still dreams of winning the Tour de France. Pain in my groin's gone. Funny how my body can produce a pain and then it disappears without me knowing anything about why I had it. It sort of mends itself.

Thoughts interrupted by a scream from Susie, who'd been searching for sellotape for Mum's birthday card. She'd found some cigarettes in a tin Dad keeps odds and ends in on the top shelf in the kitchen. A month ago he told us he'd given up and was chewing this Nicorette gum to help, though we guessed he hadn't from the occasional stink of cigarettes in the garage. We decided on war. Went down to the local toy shop and bought a packet of cigarette bangers. Stuffed a couple into the end of his remaining three fags. The packet actually had written on it 'Protect Children—Don't Make Them Breathe Your Smoke'. Carefully put the tin back on the top shelf again.

The afternoon seemed to drag on and on. Susie and I kept looking at one another and laughing. Mum and Dad knew something was up, but we didn't tell them. Just before supper Dad disappeared upstairs to the bog. A minute later the bog exploded, followed by Dad shouting a four-letter word, VERY loud. Needless to say, it was one that he keeps telling US not to use. Susie and I collapsed in laughter and Mum gave us a LOOK. After five minutes silence Dad appeared, saying nothing but sucking a mint. I'm not bad at recognizing the smell of polo and cigarette smoke, though Dad's smell seemed tinged with gunpowder.

Supper was a bit strained. Susie couldn't resist repeating something I'd told her. 'Dad, did you know that it was Sir Walter Raleigh who first brought tobacco to England in the sixteenth century, and that doctors used to think it was good for all sorts of things like gout, and head lice, and ulcers? But now the National Health Service is having to spend over £4,000,000 each week looking after people with illnesses due to smoking. Of every 1,000 people, over a lifetime, 1 will be murdered, 6 will get killed on the roads, and 250 will be killed by smoking. And what's more, it makes you impotent. Are you sure you feel all right, Dad?' So innocent, my little sister can be.

Mum was perplexed, but Dad choked on his cream topping and looked like a naughty boy. In the end he had to laugh. 'Yes, it's a filthy habit and I hope you never try it. In fact, I'll give you £200 if you haven't smoked by the time you're 21.'

I said that wasn't much compared with the £40,000 HIS smoking habit would cost over a lifetime, and he didn't need to bribe US to stop us from smoking. I'm a right hypocrite myself when I want to be. Ever since Sam's dad had bribed HIM, I'd been looking for a way to get Dad to bribe me.

Susie seemed amazed at my attitude. But there was no stopping Dad now. 'You've all the facts and it's got to be the stupidest thing to do. The worst thing is that once you've started like me, it's almost impossible to stop.' Oh God, it began to sound like another school lecture, until Susie burst into tears saying, 'You mustn't die, Dad. You still splutter and cough in the mornings, and when you smoke, we have to breathe in your fumes.'

Mum insisted we stop nagging, or he'd need a cigarette to calm his nerves. So to help, I told my latest cigarette joke. ' Q. Why does a man have a dog with no legs called Cigarette? A. Because every night he takes him out for a drag.' Dead silence. It was lucky that it was my night for the washing up.

Sunday 18th June
Raining.

Monday 19th June
Raining and school.

Tuesday 20th June
Dad's got an anti-cigarette fixation. Maybe it's because I cut a photograph of a cancerous lung out of a magazine I'd found and left it in his lunch box. Discovered it torn up in the waste-paper basket. He must feel really worried that him smoking will start us too. He sat us down after tea and read from this newspaper

article about how one in three grown-ups who smoke regularly started before 9, and that children under the age of 16 smoke 20,000,000 cigarettes and spend over two million pounds on them each week, and that by year 10 at school one in three children smoke.

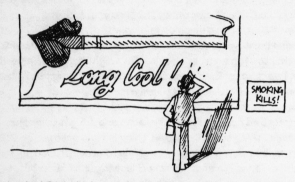

I asked Dad why he smoked, and he said it was because being addicted to nicotine was as impossible to kick as being addicted to heroin. He found he couldn't concentrate so well if he didn't smoke, and he liked the feel of the cigarette in his mouth, and the whole routine of striking a match and lighting up. You could get help to give up the addiction with nicotine patches, sprays, or gum, but it was still hard to give up. All the reasons which the person from Health Education had told us smokers give as excuses. But Dad insisted that it wasn't all his fault. After all, the advertising companies spend £100,000,000 a year telling us why we should smoke, and the government only spends £2,000,000 telling us why we shouldn't, and collecting all the lovely tax earned from cigarette sales at the same time. Apparently the government makes 8 billion pounds every year from cigarettes. No wonder they don't want to ban cigarette advertising!

Thursday 22nd June

Dad's fixation is catching. Finally couldn't stand it any longer. Told Susie that I'd tried one, and was afraid I might get hooked on it for life. Susie said that I was mad. She had tried one two years ago, and had hated it so much she had never tried again. I admitted that it would be sad to miss the £200 Dad was offering us. We went to find him—to take up his offer.

Friday 23rd June
Sally's not getting HER £200. She put her jeans through the wash with a packet of fags in them. The whole wash is nicotine stained and the washing machine has got blocked tubes. Mum's already furious with her. Instead of revising for her exams, she's been spending all her time rehearsing the school play and down the pub.

11 **Pains,** Sprains and Wheezes

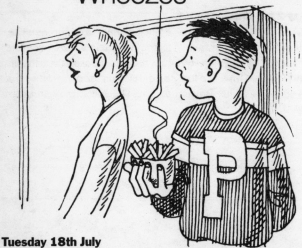

Tuesday 18th July

Only three more days to the summer holidays. Can't wait. Went to MacDonalds for some chips on the way home today, and met Cilla by accident just as I was going in. Quite embarrassing as half the school were there, and it looked as if we were together. She's obsessed with mad cow disease and BSE and wouldn't have a Big Mac.

I've fancied Cilla for ages but I don't think she knows how much. We're really good friends now, but I still don't know if I dare ask her out. She might say 'No' again. I've got to get sorted, I can't just go on fancying her from afar. I suppose the easiest thing would be to ask a girl out after getting to know her really well at a party or something. I hope this happens to me sometime. At the moment I'm still hopeless at it.

Wednesday 19th July

Two more days to the summer holidays. It's Sally's last term at school, and everyone's gone to watch her as Juliet in *Romeo* and Juliet this evening. I didn't go as I'd sat through it once already and I know enough about family feuds. They can be a bit much sometimes. Perhaps I could have learnt a bit though about what to say to Cilla. I don't know how to start saying something romantic to her without feeling a bit stupid.

I lounged at home instead, and wished I'd gone to the play. After a while, I found myself in Susie's room. She'd forgotten to lock her diary and I couldn't resist another peek. I can hardly read her handwriting. They ought to do something about that at school.

Wednesday 5th July

Mum's cross because I haven't touched my flute for three days. Said it wasn't worth me having lessons if I didn't practise. What do grown-ups have to practise? It's not fair.

Thursday 6th July

Came on today. Second one ever. I'm glad I have started, but it's a bother—especially hiding the fact from Pete, who would tease me.

Favourite supper this evening—macaroni cheese and ice-cream. Perhaps I'll become a vegetarian and stop eating poor furry animals. No more little lambs, but I know I won't be able to resist roast chicken, especially the way Mum cooks it. Told Pete I was going to be a vegetarian. He asked how I knew vegetables didn't feel just as much pain as animals. I couldn't answer that, but I can't give up eating altogether or I'll get anorexic like Jane at school.

Got soaked again running round the block with Kate, practising for the 400 metres. God seems to have forgotten about us having a summer this year. I haven't been practising enough, so I think I'll probably come last. Only a week to go.

Saturday 8th July

I'm going to have a real moan today. Pete's in a bad mood and taking it out on me. It's horrid being the youngest. My brother and sister always tease me, and when I react they do it even more. They don't seem to mind how I feel but when I tease them, they make a great fuss and shout at me. They're so bossy. They think they can tell me what to do and say. It's really humiliating in front of my friends, especially when Mum and Dad do it as well.

I'm still fed up with wearing grim, hand-me-down, cast-offs from Sally and Pete, especially as I think I'm getting fat. Last time I managed to get Mum to buy me something new, Sally teased me about trying to be 'cool'. I bet she was just the same when she was my age. And Sally and Pete are always trying to point out the advantages I have—like staying up later than they did 'when they were my age', and getting more pocket money than they did 'when they were my age', and being allowed the last lick of the cake bowl, and so on, and so on.

Sunday 9th July

Went running. Tried to get Pete to come but he stayed in bed and said he'd time me while I was gone. Wobbly Sally came instead. At least I'm faster than her. Pete was asleep when I got back. Lazy slob.

Bovril's going to the vet. No more kittens for her. Sally's got a new boyfriend, called Steve.

Wednesday 12th July

Dear diary,
Who does she think she is, Anne Frank?

All my practice was wasted! I'm sitting here with my ankle wrapped in an 'elastic' bandage. Feels more like a boa constrictor wrapped around a tree trunk.

Kate, Charlotte and me decided as it was the last practice before Sports Day, we'd do a whole lot of false starts, which was fine until Miss 'Big Bum' Court got fed up. When we finally got started we agreed that we'd all join hands and come in last together. Just before crossing the finishing line, Charlotte has to reckon she's really faster than all of us, and she let go to run over the line first. I tripped over my other foot, fell flat on my face, and twisted my ankle. What really annoys me is that, in spite of my hayfever, I'm actually faster than Charlotte but with a twisted ankle I won't get a chance to show her. I could kill her.

After the fall, I kept collapsing with pain, as my ankle wouldn't stay straight, and I cried because I thought it was broken. I had done my First Aid at Brownies so I took my shoe and sock off and gently felt around. Then I knew it wasn't actually broken, so I limped over to Miss Court.

She got Mr Jones to carry me to the sick room, with the boys saying things like, 'What will your boyfriend say?' and 'teacher's pet' and 'I hope you don't herniate yourself, Mr Jones'. Then Miss Court appeared with a packet of frozen peas from the kitchens, muttering 'RICE PAD, RICE PAD, RICE PAD'. I thought she'd gone mad until she explained that that is how she remembers what to do with bruises and sprains, and how to check that bones aren't broken. 'RICE' is for treating sprains: Rest, Ice, Compression, Elevation. 'PAD' is for checking for broken bones: Pain, Abnormal mobility, Deformity.

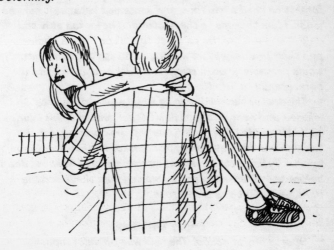

I had a quick check myself with PAD. There was lots of pain, but luckily not when Miss Court just pulled or pushed my foot, only when she twisted it. I could move it OK myself (with pain), and there didn't seem to be any worse deformity than Pete says I always have. They bandaged my ankle up with the elastic bandage (compression—and how!), told me to keep the frozen peas on it when I got home (ice), and to put my leg on a chair or something when sitting (elevation). My shoe had suddenly grown very small because of the bandage and swelling, so they found a slipper from lost property. When it was time to go home I was walking, or rather limping, but suddenly my ankle gave way so a teacher got Kate to help me.

When I got home I felt very tired and depressed. Mum was nice, treating me as if I was a child again, and she gave me my supper on the settee. Later I went to bed, but I couldn't sleep. I was in so much pain I could have screamed. I tried to find a comfortable way to lie, and finally Mum came in and gave me some paracetamol. After a while I must have fallen asleep, and when I next looked at the time it was morning.

I was ten minutes late getting up, so I jumped out of bed, forgetting I had a bad foot, and screamed because it hurt so much. Mum took me to the doctor and he looked at it and said it was bruised. He said not to walk on it for a whole day, and then gradually start walking on it with the bandage on. It would probably go on hurting for a week or two. I could take paracetamol to help the pain.

The doctor turned out to be a real expert on sports injuries, and went on about how 80 per cent of these injuries could be avoided if only everyone prepared properly for training and competition by being fit for their own individual sports, by being careful about warming up and warming down before and afterwards, and by making sure they used the right equipment and techniques.

Friday 14th July

Sports Day at school. The field was so wet, I thought it

might be postponed and then I could have run after all.
During the morning I tried to teach Kate the tactics to beat
Charlotte, as we were still cross with her for causing my
accident. We thought we might demand a drugs test on
Charlotte. She looks as if she's on steroids, anyhow. It's sad
anyone having to use drugs to win, and especially famous
people.

Sports Day wasn't postponed, and I had to sit on the wet
grass and watch and freeze. I felt sorry for Sam, as he had a
bad attack of asthma during his run and came in last. While I
was watching I kept Rachel company. She goes everywhere in
a wheelchair. She can't use her legs because of something
called Cerebral Palsy that she's had from birth. I'd never
talked to her before, but she's really nice. Must be awful for
her, never being able to run.

When the 400 metres was called I felt this kind of tension
in my stomach for Kate. It's funny how nervous I can get for
someone else. They were really close at the finish, but
Charlotte won. I had to pretend to be pleased for her, even
though my best time had been three seconds faster. As we
were sitting there, Rachel and me, we were a captive audience.
Everybody came to sympathize and then ended up telling us
about their own injuries.

John said that when he was playing football another
player had done a sliding tackle. He fell in a funny way and
twisted his ankle, which swelled up like a balloon. He had gone
to the hospital where they X-rayed it and said there was
nothing wrong. A couple of weeks later he had gone to stamp
on a friend's foot. He missed and twisted his ankle again,
and it all swelled up.

Frank had been knocked out playing goalie. The ball was
kicked towards him, he dived to smother it, and the full force
of a defender's boot hit his temple. He didn't know how long
he was out, but people told him it was half a minute. He
remembered getting up with the help of his coach, but he
staggered about all over the place and couldn't carry on

playing. Although he felt quite clear-headed at half-time, at the end of the game he couldn't remember what had happened or what the score was. When he got home he was sick and sleepy and had to go to hospital.

Football seems dangerous because then Timmy said that when HE had played in goal someone had kicked his arm instead of the ball, and then stood on it. He was taken off to hospital with it broken. The result was that he couldn't do any work, as it was his right arm, but he couldn't play football either!

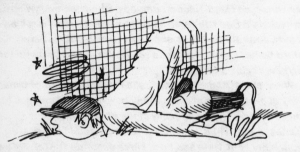

Jan had bruised her bum and broken her collar bone when SHE went over a jump and her horse didn't. She was taken to the medical tent where they put a funny bandage round her shoulders, but her own doctor had taken it off. He said that although normally one had to stop broken bones from moving for them to mend (like when Pete broke his arm), the collar bone would heal up OK by itself.

Beth said that she had been playing basketball when she had tried to dive out of the way of another girl. She had landed on her nose and had had her fingers crushed when the girl's head landed on them. The pain had made her feel dizzy and sick.

I was saved from any more by kind Mum, who came to take me home. Wish my ankle would get better.

I bet dick-head Dave didn't tell her about the time he twisted his bollocks doing a one-handed hopping windmill, and had to have THEM put into plaster. I'd read enough.

Friday 21st July

Last day of school. No one did any work. Don't know why we bother to go in.

Sam's not coming with us to France these holidays. His whole family is going to Italy, as his dad's got a conference there. Sam fancies himself as a real runner, always first or second in cross country, while Randy Jo and me hide in the pack. But on Sports Day last week he was last in the 100 metres and collapsed, wheezing horribly, till someone gave him his inhaler to puff. He uses it quite often, especially before he runs, which stops him wheezing or as he says 'getting asthma'. Sam's so brill at everything I really hate him sometimes. I showed him a leaflet about asthma that came with the stuff on hayfever from the radio station.

It said asthma is a disease of the lungs in which the muscles round the air passages get all tight. The air passages, or 'bronchioles', as the leaflet called them, get narrowed, and stop the easy flow of air into, but more especially out of, the air sacs where the oxygen in the air normally crosses into the blood. People with asthma not only get wheezy, but feel as if they are suffocating as well, which is very frightening.

Under the section 'WHAT CAUSES ATTACKS' it said:

Asthma is not infectious. It's just that the air passages in the lungs of asthmatic children are very sensitive and their narrowing can be set off by many different things. For instance, changes in the weather, particularly cold weather or strong winds; pollution; emotional strains such as excitement, or prolonged laughing; infections (colds which go to the chest); exercise (Sam's main problem) and allergy. Allergy is a special form of sensitivity in which substances which don't affect most people start attacks in those with asthma. Common things that people are allergic to include: house dust, grass pollen, and fur and skin flakes from animals.

A lot of the allergy stuff sounded just like hayfever, without the runny eyes. I'm still waiting to see what I'm allergic to (not counting my mum saying I'm allergic to hard work). The leaflet went on:

Treatment of Asthma

Present-day treatment does not cure asthma, but it usually enables children with quite severe asthma to lead a normal life. To do this they may need to take medicines during school hours. These medicines are of two different types:

(1) Treatment which the child takes when the wheezing has started. This is usually in the form of a spray called Salbutamol (Ventolin) to be breathed into the lungs. It gives immediate relief by relaxing the lung muscles and opening up the narrowed air passages.

(2) Treatment which decreases the sensitivity of the lungs to what normally sets off an attack, and so prevents the narrowing of the air passages and the resulting wheezing. This treatment may also be a medicine to be breathed in called Beclomethasone (Becotide).

If these medicines are not taken regularly and properly, severe asthma may develop.

This bit of the leaflet reminded me of the time Sam was had up in front of the head for using his inhaler, because his teacher thought he was taking drugs!

Monday 24th July

Have to seek Dad's advice on sex after all. Mr Rogers has set us homework on 'Contraception' and 'Sexually Transmitted Diseases'—disgusting—with seven sheets of questions to be answered by next term. What a way to spend the holidays—finding out about sex!

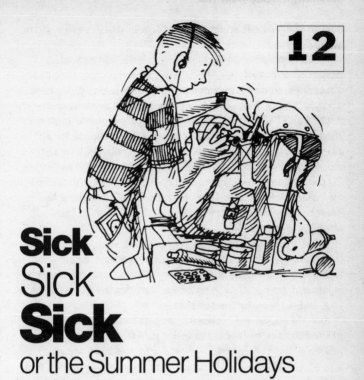

12

Sick
Sick
Sick
or the Summer Holidays

Friday 28th July

Gran's not coming camping with us after all. It didn't appeal.
She's going to Bournemouth instead. Wouldn't catch me
sharing a tent with HER. Even saved from sharing with Susie,
as Mat's coming instead of Sam, and bringing his two-man
tent.

He's lucky. He's getting two holidays, first with us while his
mum works, and then in Scotland with her, as his parents are
divorced.

Saturday 29th July

Not so sure I like holidays. Mum ordered me to pack my own
stuff. Dad said 'One case only' as he isn't having any last-

minute plastic bags under the seats, or blocking his view at the back of the car.

Did a great job—all my tapes, my heads, fishing tackle, penknife, medical dictionary, *Animal Farm* and this year's photo magazines, some other books, my zit creams, anti-perspirant spray, athletes' foot powder, my new trainers, my first-aid booklet and the first-aid kit Uncle Bob gave me last Christmas. There seemed enough in that to equip a field hospital for a disaster. It contained: a tube of Savlon, 20 swabs, 10 non-adherent Melonin dressings, 25 adhesive plasters, 3 bandages, 20 paracetamol, 10 magnesium trisilicate compound tablets for indigestion, Calamine cream, scissors and tweezers. Mum never has anything like this on holiday and you never know what's going to happen.

I didn't pack anything else. There wasn't room. Unfortunately Mum decided to check my packing. She's impossible. I had to take most of my gear out and put clothes in instead. So I stuffed the books and medicines into a plastic bag, and hid it under the car seat.

Long 'discussions' between Mum and Dad about why she needed to take 'her whole wardrobe, plus the kitchen sink'. We had to go back three times—first for Mum's bikini top which was still on the washing line, then for my swimming trunks, and finally for Susie's sleeping bag. Then we had to stop in a lay-by near Maidstone. Mat had suddenly gone silent and puked over Susie and the sleeping bags. Heard Dad mutter that we'd make Dover in three months if we were lucky.

While Mum mopped up, I looked 'motion sickness' up in my medical dictionary. No one knows its cause, but it does involve the middle part of the ear, which is to do with balance, and the eyes. Deaf mutes don't get it, and Mat was in good company— Julius Caesar, Lord Nelson, Charles Darwin and Lawrence of Arabia were all travel pukers. I wouldn't want to be the next person to stop at that lay-by.

I was sent into the chemist at Dover for travel-sick pills, instead of Susie who's still pretending her ankle's a bit wobbly.

It's fine when she wants it to be. Came out clutching packets of both Kwells and Stugeron, as the chemist didn't know whether one was better than the other. The packets said that they must be taken well in advance of travelling, and that they: 'May cause drowsiness. If affected, do not drive or operate machinery. Avoid alcoholic drink.'

The waves coming over the harbour walls persuaded Mum and Susie to try the Kwells and Mat the Stugeron. Dad doesn't get seasick, and I KNEW it wouldn't happen to me. I may be a hypochondriac but I'm not a weakling. Anyway, the instructions that came with the pills gave hints to help avoid travel sickness:

At Sea
When possible, stay on deck and look at the horizon. Keep away from diesel and galley smells. Avoid rich and fatty foods. If below decks, lie face down with eyes closed.

On the road
If possible, look forward into the distance. Try to ensure children can see out of windows. Avoid reading while in motion. Travel by daylight if possible. Ensure fresh air and no fumes. Avoid rich and fatty foods.

On the boat had chips, bacon, eggs and sausages with Mat and Susie. Wasted mine. It all ended up feeding the seagulls in the Channel while Mat and Susie sneaked off and won the jackpot on the fruit machines. Will have to take the seasick pills next time, or persuade Dad to go through the tunnel.

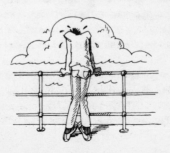

Sunday 30th July

This is being written in a wet T-shirt (motto 'DON'T SIT ON THE GRASS—SMOKE IT') in a soggy sleeping bag, in a soaking tent, in a French mud patch called a camping site, somewhere in Brittany. Might just as well be in our back garden. Desperate for a pee. Don't know where to go. It's already daylight so can't go outside and let go. I'm hungry after the sea pukes. Mat's still asleep, exhausted by talking most of the night about his parents and what it was like when they got divorced.

He said it was terrible at first—all the shouting and arguing. He'd wondered whether it was something he'd done wrong, but it obviously wasn't. Then he'd worried that if they didn't love one another, perhaps they didn't love him either. When his dad finally left, Mat had begun wetting his bed every night, but he didn't any more (was glad to hear that!). He said that although separated parents weren't what he would choose to have, it was better than having parents who live together but don't speak to each other, or have violent arguments.

Luckily, Mat's divorced parents still talk to one another and are friendly, except over the phone sometimes discussing arrangements for meeting. One of the bad things was that he never felt he saw enough of his dad, but he also worried about his mum being lonely when he was away or staying with his dad. It was nice though, he said, to be living in the same house, so that all the other things that he was used to, since as far back as he could remember, were still there and hadn't changed. Some of the other good things were having two rooms of his own, in two separate places, two birthday parties, two Christmases, and lots of presents. One of the best things was that his dad and step-mum had had another baby boy he really liked.

If this had been the only thing that I'd heard about parents getting divorced, I think I'd have had a word with my own, but it seems to have been worse for some of my other friends. God, I'm desperate. I'll burst if I don't find a pissary somewhere.

Saturday 5th August

Too depressed to write for a week. Rain, rain, rain, rain, rain. I've seen the inside of more churches than the Pope. Dead boring. How it's 'good for you' I don't know. I'm not even holy, just an existential agnostic Marxist, devoted to dialectical materialism—and my own body.

It wasn't good for Susie. In the last cathedral she was lighting up a candle to the Patron Saint of Animals, or someone, and she turned round to find an old man with his mackintosh open, flashing his knob. Said her first reaction was 'yugh', not at what he was doing, but at the actual thing itself. It looked so puny and wrinkled. She was also surprised and shocked (it's not the sort of thing one normally expects in a cathedral), but then she thought, be smart, don't scream or cry or run away. That's what pervs want you to do. Just be cool and leave, so she walked away. The guy must have been really miffed.

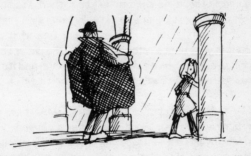

Sunday 6th August

Poor Susie. Flashed at yesterday, the pukes and runs today. Wonder if it's all psychological? She said it was bad enough getting the runs at the best of times, but on a holiday camp site with the lavs all made of concrete and smelling of stale pee! She wants to go home. Wish she would, she's becoming a real pain.

Dad said it was from eating too many peaches. Mat said it was the water. I think it was all in her mind. But Mum said the doctor told her that people often get an upset tummy when abroad on holiday owing to coming in contact with new bugs.

She said it wasn't usually serious, only lasted a couple of days, and normally got better without having to spend money on medicines. Instead, Susie had to stop eating and drink lots of clear fluids, like water or weak fruit juices, a little at a time so that she didn't puke up again.

The medical dictionary said it was called different names in different parts of the world: Hong Kong Dog, Delhi Belly, Aztec Two-Step, Rangoon Runs. I don't think Susie's was much like these. More like 'Silly Susie's Sloppy French Shits'. Hope it's cholera.

Monday 7th August

No sleep. Susie tripped over our tent pegs all last night. Wonder if she made it to the lavs? She gave us the details this morning over coffee and croissants.

She said she had had a really heavy feeling in her arms and legs, dead annoying because she couldn't be bothered to think or do anything. The worst thing was actually being sick. And having the runs meant you were worrying all the time whether you would do it in your pants before you got to the lav, or before you had finished puking. She said her bum was sore, and itched, but Mum had given her my Savlon cream to put on it which had helped.

SUNNY DAY! At last a chance to get my HE-MAN tan. Perhaps my acne will improve too. It might even disappear altogether! Mutiny at Dad's suggestion of going to local nudist beach. I'm not taking all MY clothes off. Susie, who has almost NOTHING, refuses to go topless even. Wish Mum would refuse as well. She might have a bit of consideration for Mat.

Tuesday 8th August

Agggggh—the agony. Feels like a thousand needles being shoved about under my skin, or as though boiling water had been poured all over me removing my skin. Can't bear the touch of anything. Even if Cilla put her naked body next to mine I'd scream for her to go away. None of me's brown, just bright red like an over-cooked tomato.

I'm lying in my tent wearing Calamine cream and nothing else. Everyone else is in the sun. Clever me. Didn't listen to Mum when she said put some lotion on and take it easy in the sun. It didn't feel hot. I spent the whole day displaying my muscles, with only my swimming trunks on. (At least THAT bit of me is spared. It's the only white painless part left. I'm even gladder we refused to go to the nudist beach.) Wasn't till evening my skin caught fire.

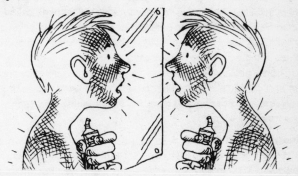

Took some paracetamol for the pain. Smart-arse Susie read out the French notice on the camp board. It said:

ATTENTION!
IL EST TRÈS DANGEREUX DE RESTER AU SOLEIL . . .

She waited till Mat was around to impress him with her translation: 'Look out, it is very dangerous to lie around in the sun for long periods of time. Only expose your skin to the sun for short periods, and particularly avoid the middle of the day when the sun is strongest. Use appropriate sun tan lotions (high block), especially if you have fair and sensitive skin. Wear a hat to protect your head from direct sunlight. Too much sun may lead to skin cancer.'

Wednesday 9th August
WORSE . . . weepy blisters everywhere and bits of skin coming off. Mum says it's the outside layer only. When it gets burnt, all

the cells in this layer die and are removed by what's called 'serous' fluid. Luckily if the burns are not too deep, the body just grows a new layer of skin to take its place. I'm busy drinking lots of coke to make up for all the wet coming off me (including the sweat!), and eating tons of french bread, butter, and paté, with fruit and chocolate and sloppy cheeses, to help my poor old body make itself up.

Medical dictionary says that getting brown is when cells in the skin called 'melanocytes' start making a pigment called 'melanin', which filters the sunlight and stops it from being able to burn the skin. Hope there'll be a chance for my melanocytes to get going before the next downpour.

Susie's getting her own back for my lack of sympathy over her 'French Shits'—poking her mug into the tent, not asking me how I am, just staring and bursting out laughing, and then disappearing with Mat.

Thursday 10th August

Late night discussion, with bugs smashing around the tent. Susie and Mat on about divorce again. Susie was horrified when Mat said that nowadays more than one in three marriages ends in divorce, and that half the children of these broken marriages lose contact with one of their parents. He also said that a common effect on children was they started to do worse at school. That's what happened to him. I wonder if that's what will happen to the Royals?—though they don't have many brains to start with.

Susie said that her friend Pam's parents were divorced and she hardly saw her dad, but Pam felt she had really grown away from him completely and although he was her biological father, she didn't actually like him much. She knew he wanted to see her more, but it was a 'duty' for her, and a real drag having to leave her friends and go somewhere where she didn't know anybody. What's more, everyone thought she should be good friends with her step-sister, who got on her nerves 90 per cent of the time.

This wasn't Mat's experience, but it was different for everybody. All his friends whose parents were having 'problems' or getting divorced came to him, because they thought he would know what they were going through—the arguments, the door-slamming, the accusations, the tears, the feeling it was all their fault, the long silences, the guilt, the resentment.

Blisters better. Even a tinge of brown, but still very cautious about the sun. Looking forward to going home. Susie said she wished I'd go now.

Friday 11th August

Susie's retribution. She and Mat are covered with plague. Probably mosquito bites. Hope they get malaria. Offered my Savlon (almost all used up on Susie's bum) and Calamine in return for an ice-cream from their fruit machine winnings. Medical dictionary said no chance of malaria. These mosquitoes don't carry it. Itching and red bumps (Mum's got them too) are the body reacting to the bugs' saliva which they inject when they bite.

Saturday 12th August

Home, loaded with duty-free fags which Dad says are 'for someone at work'! Postcard from Cilla. She's brown all over. Take back what I said about rejecting her naked body.

Bovril's fleas leapt up to greet us. Popped her into a string bag and sprayed her all over with de-fleaing stuff—another enemy for life.

13

Future **Fears**

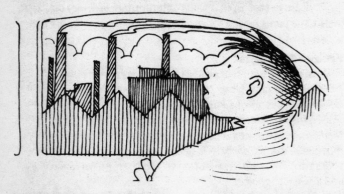

Tuesday 5th September

Back to school today. Cilla's really brown. DETERMINED to be her boyfriend.

Wednesday 6th September

Only been back a day and they're already going on about GCSEs and tests. Seems nothing else is going to matter from now. We've been given a timetable for the term, which looks horrific, and a note to say that our exercise books mustn't have any graffiti on them. They're becoming just like policemen—perhaps they think that otherwise computer games will rule over us. Mum and Dad have to sign a homework diary and say what THEY think about our work.

Monday 11th September

Yesterday was Sam's birthday treat. He's 15. Was too wiped out to write last night after three hundred and sixty miles in his dad's BMW and three hours at a rad amusement park. Sam,

Randy Jo, Mat, and myself. It was more fun than usual, as I took car-sick pills for the journey and was able to stand up to Sam's dad's driving (almost as bad as Mum's). I could go on the Nemesis, Multiversion Roller Coaster, where you end up sitting on your head as you go over the top completely hanging in suspension, without a whiff of throwing up. There were long queues for everything, but we took it in turns waiting while the others went off for hamburgers and to pee.

Passed through Birmingham on the way—really depressing, endless rows of dirty chimneys polluting the atmosphere. Sam's dad said that smoking chimneys weren't the only environmental problem. We were back to tobacco again. In Third World countries, to clear the land to grow the tobacco for just 300 fags, one tree is being cut down; and worldwide, six million hectares of farmland, which could feed 20 million people, was being used to grow tobacco. As far as pollution is concerned, every day in the United Kingdom smokers throw away 20 million fag packets and 300 million butts.

Unemployment is a major health problem as well. Doctors were just beginning to realize that unemployment causes not only feelings of helplessness and depression, and attempted suicide (the risk of this last was increased by nine times in the unemployed) but also physical problems like heart and lung diseases.

I felt really depressed. It's something I worry about a lot, especially now Sally's failed her exams, doesn't have a job, and doesn't know what to do. It must be really awful not to have a job, especially if you're young and there looks as if there's no hope. Nearly three million are unemployed, and though they say the figure is going down, it doesn't feel as though it is. I can understand someone without a job wanting to do themselves in. The government keeps talking about the 'feel-good factor', though I don't know where it is, especially if Dad loses his job. Maybe I'll have to get a job in another country now we're in Europe.

Sam's more worried about war, and what is going on in

Bosnia. He's really upset about all the money spent on tanks and planes, when it could be used to feed starving people. Randy Jo said he thought it would be a good idea if there WAS a war as it would get rid of unemployment, either by killing us all or by us all having to fight in the army. He thinks the last world war looks really great from the TV series. This daft idea made Sam's dad swerve across the road nearly crashing into the back of a huge transporter lorry carrying Japanese cars. He just missed it. When he recovered a bit he said the world wasn't all depressing—at least they'd ended apartheid in South Africa.

Now to top it all we've got BSE, thanks to the Government's stupidity in allowing sheep to be fed to cows. It just ain't natural, even I know that. Sam says his Dad says it's all due to things called prions (never heard of them!).

Wednesday 20th September

Got back all the work I'd done for Mr Rogers over the summer holidays. Mine was the best in the class, but all my friends wanted to know how I came to know so much about sexually transmitted diseases. Mainly from my dad—but didn't let on. They said was it going to France for my holidays? I said 'Yes' because actually it was the hours lying in sunburnt agony in my tent, reading a medical dictionary. But I left that bit out.

You'd better learn this or there will be a lot of unwanted Paynes in the world!

Name Peter Payne

CONTRACEPTION

1. **Before an egg can grow into a fully-formed baby it must be**
   Fertilized ✓

2. **How many eggs are released each month?** Two or three *Usually one*

3. **How many sperms are contained in an average ejaculation?**
   100,000,000 ✓

4. **How many sperms are needed to fertilize one egg?** One ✓

5. **How long can sperm live inside a woman's body?** About three days

6. **How can a woman get pregnant if a man does not reach a climax (ejaculate)?** She can't *Men leak sperm even before they ejaculate*

7. **What does contraception mean?** Ways of stopping getting pregnant when making love

8. **What are the chances of a girl getting pregnant if she has sexual intercourse once without contraception 14 days before her next period?** Don't know. 1 in 3 chance - and you wouldn't cross the road if there was a 1 in 3 chance of getting killed would you?

9. **What is a condom?** It's like a long rubber balloon you put on your penis before making love

10. **Give another name for a condom:** Rubber, Durex, sheath, Johnny, French letter, Japanese wrinkle?

11. **How do condoms work?** Stop the sperm getting spilt into the woman's vagina

12. **Are condoms reliable?** Yes

13. **What are the advantages of condoms?** Easy to use. Easy to keep around if you suddenly want to make love. Cheap, easy to buy anywhere, everybody knows about them. and they protect against sexually transmitted diseases, including AIDS, and cervical cancer.

14. **What is an oral contraceptive?** A hormone pill that women swallow

15. **How does the Pill work?** Kills the egg - No - most stop the ova from being released from the ovary. A few stop the fertilized egg from being implanted.

16. **How reliable is the Pill?** Most reliable method available at the moment

17. **What are the disadvantages of the Pill?** Don't know It interferes with women's hormones. You have to see a doctor to get it. It also doesn't protect you against getting AIDS and other STDs.

18. **What is the proper name for the withdrawal method?** Coitus Interruptus

19. **Is the withdrawal method a reliable method of contraception?** It's OK No - it's very unreliable - but better than nothing

20. **How does the rhythm or natural method work?** By not having sex near the time when the egg is released (called ovulation)

21. **Is the rhythm method very reliable?** ~~Yes~~ No, it's not a safe method. A lot of people get pregnant this way because ―――――

22. **What are the disadvantages of the rhythm method?** ~~Don't know~~ it's very difficult to know when ovulation actually occurs, and people often want to make love when it's not a safe time

23. **What is an IUD?** Intra-uterine device

24. **Is an IUD reliable?** Yes ✓

25. **How does an IUD work?** Stops fertilized egg from becoming implanted in the womb ✓

26. **Are there any disadvantages in using an IUD?** Yes – falls out all the time. Sometimes, but main problem is risk of infection in young women

27. **Give another word for a diaphragm:** Cap ✓

28. **How is a diaphragm used?** It's put into the vagina before making love and covers the cervix to stop the sperm reaching the ovum ✓

29. **Is the diaphragm method safe?** Yes Hope so I think my mum uses it

30. **What are the advantages of the diaphragm?** Don't know. Never tried it. Safe, protects against some STDs, doesn't interfere with the woman's hormones

31. **Are there any disadvantages to using a diaphragm?** Don't know. Always have to remember to put it in before making love.

32. **What is a spermicidal chemical?** *kills sperms dead* ✓

33. **How are spermicidal chemicals used?** *Should be used with diaphragms and condoms.* ✓

34. **Are spermicidal chemicals safe?** *No, not on their own* ✓

35. **What is involved in sterilization?** *The fallopian tubes in the woman or the spermatic cords in the man are cut and/or tied* ✓

36. **Is sterilization a reliable method of contraception?**
Yes if the docter does it right ✓

37. **Are there any disadvantages to sterilization?** *No. Yes - it's difficult to change your mind if you want to have babies later.*

DISEASES ASSOCIATED WITH SEX

1. **What does STD stand for?** *Sexually transmitted disease*

2. **Give the names of 4 STDs**
   (a) *AIDS*   (b) *Gonorrhea*   (c) *Pubic lice*   (d) *Vaginal + Penile warts*

3. **Can they be transmitted by**
   (a) Lavatory seats *Probably No*
   (b) Kissing *No* ✓
   (c) French kissing *Unlikely* ✓
   (d) Vaginal intercourse *Yes* ✓
   (e) Holding hands *No* ✓

(f) Anal intercourse _Yes._ ✓

(g) Masturbation _NO_ ✓

4. What causes the following sexually transmitted diseases?

(a) Acquired Immune Deficiency Syndrome (AIDS)
Rampant virus. ✓ _HIV_

(b) Syphilis _A micro thing - called a spirochaete_

(c) Non-specific urethritis (NSU) _A sort of bacteria_ ✓

(d) Thrush _A kind of mushroom   a yeast_

(e) Vaginal and penile warts _Virus_ ✓

(f) Herpes _Herpes simplex virus_ ✓

(g) Crabs _Lice that live in the pubic hair_ ✓
Yes, but different from the head ones

(h) Gonorrhoea _Don't know   a bacteria_

5. AIDS

How do you know you have it? _You feel incredibly ill and weak - get lumps in your glands all over your body._ _but you can carry the virus and be infectious but not be ill yourself_

How can you treat it? _You can't_

How can you reduce the risk of getting it? _Don't sleep around. Don't be a drug addict. Use condoms for sex. One partner only is safest_

What happens if you don't treat it? _You die - but not everyone does._ _and, as you say above, there's no treatment_

6. Gonorrhoea

How do you know you have it? _You get pus coming out of your penis. Women get a discharge from their vagina_

How can you treat it? With penicillin – invented by Alexander Fleming – wonder if he had it?

7. Thrush

How do you know you have it? You have little mushrooms and things. You get a red itchy penis or vagina. It's not always a sexually transmitted disease.

How can you treat it? Go to a clinic or to your G.P. – it's very easily treated with a cream

How can you reduce the risk of getting it? Don't know It's very common and usually not a problem

What happens if you don't treat it? Don't know You just stay itchy!

8. Vaginal and Penile Warts

How do you know you have them? You can see them ✓

How can you treat them? You can pick them off No – there's a special paint you can get from your doctor

How can you reduce the risk of getting them? Don't have sex with someone who has them

What happens if you don't treat them? Nothing much but nobody wants to know you.

9. Herpes

How do you know you have it? You get a cold sore of the penis or vagina

How can you treat it? No treatment ✗ Joke – whats the difference between herpes and love ∑

Answer - herpes is forever) Not a joking
matter

How can you reduce the risk of getting it? _Not sleeping with_
anyone who's got it

What happens if you don't treat it? _Pops up every now and_
then

10. Non-specific urethritis (NSU)

How do you know you have it? _It hurts when you pee_
Women often don't know they've got it
but can pass it on.

How can you treat it? _No sex or alcohol for 3 weeks!_
and take an antibiotic

How can you reduce the risk of getting it? _Don't have sex with_
Someone who has it - and using Japanese
Wrinkles Does this mean condoms? If so ✓

What happens if you don't treat it? _Goes on hurting and_
you pass it on

11. Which of the following is correct about the virus which causes AIDS?

(a) It is only a homosexual disease _Mostly Not true._
Most cases in the world are caught by sex
between men and women - although most cases
in the UK so far are from sex between men and
men.

(b) Men and women can catch it _True_ ✓

(c) There is no real danger from it _False_ ✓

(d) More than 25,000 people in Britain have it _True I hope_
I'm not one of them so do I!

(e) At the moment the disease is incurable _True_ ✓

(f) Drug addicts are at increased risk _True_ ✓

(g) Using condoms helps prevent getting it. _True_ ✓

(h) Having sex with lots of people makes you more likely to get it

True

12. Crabs—Pubic lice

How do you know you have them? *You get itchy round your balls. Girls get itchy in their pubic hair.*

How can you treat them? *Use a special lotion from the chemist called Durbac – or burn them with a lighter* Definitely not. ~~would be very painful~~.

How can you reduce the risk of getting them? *Don't sleep with anyone who has them.*

What happens if you don't treat them? *You get more and more of them.*

13. What should you do if you think that you might have a sexually transmitted disease?

Go to your doctor or to a special clinic for sexually transmitted diseases in a hospital.

Very good.

Thursday 21st September

Depressed. Asked Cilla to the cinema and she said 'No'. I curled up inside. Why does it hurt so?

Don't think my ego can take it. Sam got the nomination for class rep on the school council instead of me.

Friday 22nd September

Sticking in my monitoring form from previous week—praise from Mum at last!

Monitoring Form

Homework and planning for week's work

Explain what will happen in diagram of energy changes and particles
Mystery plays
Who was most responsible for Eva's death?
Find out why castles declined
Write out arguments for and against private schools

Student's comments and targets

(records of achievements made this week, problems encountered, targets set for the future, items to remember, etc.)

Aim to work HARDER in some classes. Be seen to make an effort (don't chat . . .!). Try harder in PE. Pleased with my knowledge about sex.

Teacher's comments

Pete has done some good work this week, especially in maths. I'm concerned that he was late handing in his first English assignment. He tends to leave some homework until the last minute.

Parents' comments

We are pleased with him. He seems to be making progress. We are particularly interested in how he knows so much about sex.

Wish mum had left the sex bit out.

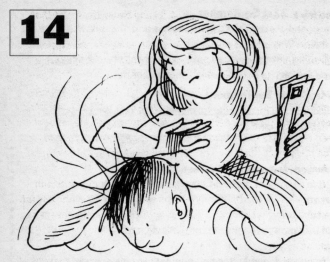

14

Little and **Large**

Tuesday 26th September

Susie's mad at me because I opened one of her letters 'by mistake'. Like doing that—gives me a thrill. It was from someone who writes the agony page for *Teenage Weekly*—the next best thing to *Sugar*. Seems Susie must have written to her about being overweight. Can't really see why. It said:

Agony Column
Teenage Weekly
Wigmore Road
London WC1

Dear Susie
   Thank you for your letter.
   You say that you are overweight, always have been, and having

recently lost 2 kilos you have put 1.5 kilos back. You insist that you are constantly trying to lose weight!

You also write that some of your family are unsympathetic, your brother calling you a hippopotamus and your father saying you don't eat enough to keep a mouse alive.

All these problems are very common, but fortunately people come in all shapes and sizes. Our height and weight only become problems when we decide we don't like the way we are, especially when we get teased by people who are stupid enough to enjoy it. Such people are hurtful and play on our weaknesses. They make us feel helpless and inadequate.

It is unfair that some people seem to eat huge amounts and stay very thin, and other people seem to eat very little and get fat. The trouble is that nobody knows exactly why this is. I always say that if you are putting on too much weight, then you are eating too much for YOU.

However, it doesn't seem as though you are very overweight at 52 kilos, as you can see from the charts of normal weights and heights of girls and boys that I have enclosed for you.

GIRLS

AGE	WEIGHT (kgs)			HEIGHT (cms)		
	Low Normal	Middle	High Normal	Low Normal	Middle	High Normal
10 yrs	24	33	50	126	139	151
11 yrs	26	37	55	130	144	158
12 yrs	29	40	60	135	150	164
13 yrs	33	45	65	142	155	170
14 yrs	37	50	70	147	160	173
15 yrs	40	54	74	150	162	175
16 yrs	43	56	76	151	163	176
17 yrs	44	57	77	152	164	176
18 yrs	45	58	78	152	164	176

BOYS

AGE	WEIGHT (kgs)			HEIGHT (cms)		
	Low Normal	Middle	High Normal	Low Normal	Middle	High Normal
10 yrs	24	31	46	126	139	151
11 yrs	25	34	52	130	143	157
12 yrs	28	38	57	134	147	163
13 yrs	30	43	65	140	155	171
14 yrs	35	49	72	146	162	179
15 yrs	39	55	80	153	169	185
16 yrs	44	60	85	158	173	188
17 yrs	48	64	88	161	175	190
18 yrs	51	66	90	165	176	190

Even if you are above or below this range, it doesn't mean anything is wrong with you. But if you are very much above or below, you ought to talk to someone about it.

It is quite common for girls of about your age to put on a bit of weight, and some people refer to this as 'puppy fat'. It is best to try not to get TOO fat, so that you will feel less self-conscious and enjoy doing things more. Also we know that fat grown-ups do have more health problems.

It has become fashionable for girls to think they should be very thin. Sometimes this goes too far and they don't know when to stop dieting. They THINK of themselves as fat even though they are extremely thin. This can lead to a problem called 'Anorexia Nervosa' where girls almost starve themselves to death.

I have enclosed some bits from letters that other people have written to me about these worries to show that you are not alone. I am also sending you some sensible eating hints which people have found useful.

Don't let your family get you down. Tell your brother that boys can just as easily become hippopotamuses as girls.

Yours sincerely

Chere Vainer

What people have said about being fat and thin
and some of my answers
Chere Vainer

I'm ten and a half stone and overweight, and have been since I was 10. I used to be called 'bubble, fatty, and big bum' and they said that when I ran 'there was an earth tremor'. I had a few friends but even they used to call me names behind my back. I'm hoping to get to nine stone, and then I can go to discos and enjoy myself, but I am uncertain what my right weight should be. Can you help me please? I've asked my mum but she said it didn't matter to her whether I was overweight or not.

Answer: Your mum's right. You're still you, whatever your weight. But there are ways she could help you to lose a little. I'm sending you a diet sheet and a weight chart. Show them to her and try to plan some meals together. Also, try taking more exercise, like biking to school and back. Fill in the chart to help you see whether you've lost weight.

My problem is that I am slightly overweight. I've had it since I was born, and it's not because I eat too much or don't take enough exercise. As I am tallish, my big stomach doesn't show so much especially if I wear baggy clothes. I think that it is harder for males to diet than for females. Is this true? I don't think I can help my build and I have tried dieting, but it's no good.

Answer: You can't blame your sex. It's hard for everybody to lose weight. The main thing is that you must really want to. But it doesn't sound as if you have much of a problem if you eat a healthy diet and exercise!

I am overweight though I don't eat too much. It's not really my weight that I think is the problem, more that I've got fat in all the wrong places. My legs look fat, especially my thighs, but everything else is all right. To rub salt into the wound, all my friends are slim and pretty with feminine curves. I suppose if I was a boy it would be different.

Answer: Boys and society like girls to be slim, so of course girls want to be like the models that they see all the time on television.

Don't care so much about what other people think. It's what you think of yourself that counts in the long run.

I think that I'm overweight because I eat too many sweets, but I can't stop eating them. I've tried eating the right kinds of food and lost a bit of weight, but not enough. I've tried exercise and my body ached so I couldn't do any more. I've tried everything possible but it just makes me more depressed. Last week I even bought some laxatives, but they didn't do anything. I've tried making myself sick, but it wouldn't come up.

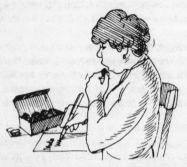

Answer: Starving, or using laxatives, or making yourself sick is DANGEROUS. Doing these things can make you anorexic. Try eating sweets on only one day of the week. When you get the craving on other days, try a carrot or an apple instead. If you find yourself lured into sweet shops then try asking for a packet of peanuts or raisins instead of sweets.

I am too thin. I was fat when I was young, but when I was about 10 I got thinner. I get called a lanky streak of bacon. How can I put on weight and be like Arny Schwarzenegger?
Answer: Not everyone finds the Schwarzenegger look attractive— me for one. Some people do find it difficult to put on weight. It's probably just the way you're made. Look on the bright side. It's generally healthier to be thin than fat.

My weight problem is that I am too thin—especially in the legs. I've had this all my life, and so has my dad. People call me 'matchstick man' and ask if they can use me to light their cigarettes. I don't care so much now as I've taken up squash and have become bigger all over. I'd rather be thin than fat. Is this right?

Answer: There is no 'right'—thin or fat. It sounds as though the size you are is right for you—like your dad whom you inherited it from. Take no notice of people making jokes. It's their own lack of self-confidence that makes them do it. We ALL have our weak points and for some people this is having to make jokes at other people's expense.

When I wear a tight skirt I get teased and called 'fatty'. My best friend says I'm not, but I feel fat. When I look in the mirror it's depressing, and when I go shopping with my friend all the nice things fit HER and are too small for ME. Why don't they make nice clothes in bigger sizes?

Answer: Shop around. Many shops do have clothes of larger sizes. In many ways you're lucky. I find the average sizes get sold out immediately.

I see myself as being different from other boys of the same age. In my eyes I am short and tubby, whereas everyone else seems tall and slim. When it comes to games I hate it. As we walk out to the sports field we have to pass the girls playing tennis. Most of them have already become mature, with breasts and things. I think that they look down on me. If one of them misses a tennis ball and laughs, I think they're laughing at me. The running track is worst. I can't run to save my life with my short fat legs, and people offer to buy me a clockwork tortoise to train with.

Answer: Fortunately we ARE all different from one another. But don't give up hope of getting taller and slimmer. When you reach puberty you may have the last laugh as some boys grow a foot in a year.

What people have said about being too tall or too short
and some of my answers
Chere Vainer

I have the problem of being too small. It first came to prominence two years ago when I was 13. I am very keen on sport and tried for the school football team. My favourite position is central defence because I like tackling players, but I wasn't picked for the first few matches. The rest of the team got at me for being too small and causing us to lose our training matches because the ball was being lobbed over my head. I was dropped, but then the player who replaced me was so terrible that I got my place back.

Answer: *As you've discovered, like many things in life, it's not your size that matters, it's the way that you use it.*

I am too tall for my age. Some people think I'm 18 and call me 'lanky'.

Answer: *Teenagers grow at different times, according to when they start and finish going through puberty. Soon all your friends will grow too, and you may want to be even taller!*

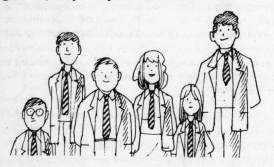

My mother took me to see the doctor because I'm very small. He said that in my case it is because all my family are small. I've always been small and people call me 'shrimpy' and 'half-pint'. People say smoking stunts your growth but I don't smoke. I've tried putting on high heels, but they make me look stupid and are just uncomfortable. It gets on my nerves when I'm buying clothes and when I buy trousers I end up by cutting off half the legs.

Answer: *Think of the advantages. You will save money when you're older as you'll be able to buy children's clothes. Think how much better being half-pint is than being quarter-pint. It's all comparative.*

I think I am too tall and get depressed about it when people call me a beanpole. When I was 11 I was short, but now I've shot up and don't even fit properly into my bed. I don't like being tall, but my dad wants me to become a policeman, and if I was short they wouldn't have me. I suppose there are some advantages. At football you can see over everyone, and having long arms helps me to play basketball.

Answer: Get your parents to buy you a double bed so that you can fit your feet in. It'll come in useful later in life.

I'm called 'titch' and 'midget', and I think I'm small because I was born prematurely. When I came to secondary school we were shown around the first day and had a woodwork lesson, and I was embarrassed because I couldn't see over the top of the bench. Because I'm small in height it makes me feel small in character. I tend to be quiet, so people say I haven't got much confidence in myself. I always find it much easier talking to someone the same size as me.

Answer: Most people who are born prematurely will end up a perfectly normal height. Concentrate on all your good points and this will make you feel more confident. Being more confident will make you FEEL bigger. Just because people are big doesn't mean that they are better.

I am so small that some people have suggested that I make a career of being a garden gnome.

Answer: Well don't—make a career out of being you, instead. Many of my friends who consider themselves 'small' develop a devastating list of cutting replies to this kind of remark. Try making some up, ready for next time.

I'm too small and I've had this problem since I was 5. I get teased and bullied, and cannot get into a '15' film without my birth certificate. When I'm in crowds, people look down on me and joke about it—even people I don't know. I laugh, but inside I get really upset. I can't wear Calvin Kleins because they don't fit me. People think that I'm younger than I am and I don't like that. I read about some children being small because they lack something called 'growth hormone'. Could this be my problem?

Answer: Growth hormone deficiency causes smallness in about 1 in 4,000 children. If you're worried I would suggest you see your family doctor and discuss it.

Susie said I ought to keep a copy of the eating hints as she thinks I'm getting a bit fat myself. The cheek. It's not true.

ARE YOU WHAT YOU EAT?
Yes—you are!

SO WHAT DO YOU KNOW ABOUT WHAT YOU'RE EATING?

1. Which food is the most concentrated source of energy?
(a) fat
(b) protein
(c) sugar
(d) alcohol
(e) dietary fibre

2. Which is the most easily available source of food energy?
a) vitamins
b) fat
c) carbohydrate
d) protein

3. If you eat too much meat, what does it get converted to?
a) muscle
b) faeces (shit)
c) fat
d) energy

4. Taking large amounts of vitamin tablets:
a) Can replace meals?
b) Can be dangerous?
c) Is necessary in addition to a good diet?

5. Which of the following does not contain carbohydrate?
a) jam
b) bread
c) milk
d) butter

6. Which of these is not high in fat?
a) lean red meat
b) fruit
c) bread and potatoes
d) cheese
e) none of these

7. Which take-away foods are low in fat?
a) hamburger without chips
b) ham and cheese sandwich
c) fish and chips
d) none of these

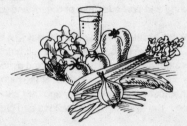

Answers
1. a
2. c
3. c
4. b
5. d
6. b and c
7. d

So what is a good diet? Most magazines, parents, and health freaks go on and on about what you should and shouldn't eat. But no one really knows exactly. What people do know is that HOW MUCH you eat of different foods is just as important as WHAT you eat. It's a matter of balance.

Throughout the world, people eat all sorts of different diets and most of them are OK as far as balance is concerned. But many people in many parts of the world are not getting ENOUGH food to give them enough energy to do what they need to do. This is what you ought to be concerned about: eating enough food to keep your energy up. You also need to get enough of some basic essentials (around fifty of them) to make sure you keep healthy.

No one food contains everything you need, so here are some very general 'goods' and 'bads'.

The basics of a good diet

- fruit, vegetables and salad: gut on these
- bread, cereals and potatoes: good fillers to stop you feeling hungry
- meat and dairy foods: choose carefully to avoid fat—fatty meat and hard cheeses are FULL of fat
- fish is fine
- oils, butter, margarine and spreads: less of these, and you'll eat less fat
- salt and sugar: you get all the salt you need per day just by eating bread and cereals, so you're probably eating far too much salt. There are natural sugars in fruit which are good and delicious. Stick with these and stay away from too much of the highly refined sugars (the stuff that looks like white sand, and that's in all the things you crave for!—the Mars bars, candy floss and chocolate cake).

Recommended Daily Amounts of Food Energy at Different Ages

AGE		ENERGY IN CALORIES
	BOYS & MEN	
9–11 years		2280
12–14 years		2640
15–17 years		2880
18–54 years	lazing	2510
	moderately active	2900
	very active	3350
	GIRLS & WOMEN	
9–11 years		2050
12–14 years		2150
15–17 years		2150
18–54 years	most occupations	2150
	very active	2500

FOOD	Calories
An Apple	50
Bacon (2 rashers)	160
A Banana	80
Baked Beans—1 portion	150
A Biscuit—chocolate	50
—wafer	100
—custard cream	60
Bread—1 slice	100
Bread/Butter/Jam	250
Butter 30 gm	210
Cakes—choc roll	120
—chelsea bun	255
—doughnut	125
—apple pie	210
—cream slice	250
—jam tart	105
A Carrot	20
Cereal—1 portion	130
Chicken Nuggets—1 portion	270
Chips—1 portion	440
Chocolate Bar	315
Crisps—1 packet	135
Cucumber—1 portion	12
Drinks—coca-cola	130
—diet pepsi	0
—fruit drinks	85
—milk shakes	365
—tea (milk & sugar)	40
Fish—1 portion	460
Hamburgers	
Big Mac	555
Standard	250
Ice Cream—a choc ice	130
—a cone	100
An Iced Lolly	55
A Lamb Chop	175
Milk—1 pint	370

Milk—1 pint skimmed	200
An Orange	50
A Pizza	
10" thin & crispy cheese and tomato	610
10" deep pan pepperoni	1585!
A Potato—jacket	170
—jacket plus butter	255
Sausages—2 pork	370
Steak—1 lean portion	300
A Tangerine	20
A Yoghurt—plain	75
—fruit	130

Wednesday 27th September

Asked Cilla to the pictures. Help! She said, 'YES'.

Sunday 1st October

Not going to wash my hand for a week. It was holding Cilla's for the last twenty minutes of the film. SUCCESS AT LAST!

Wart-Hogs and Odious Odours from Orifices

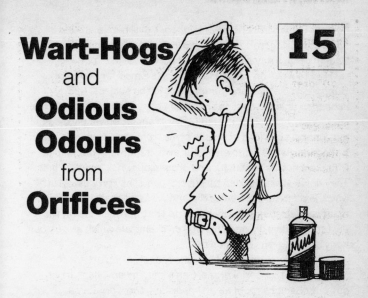

15

Tuesday 3rd October

Teachers are like parents. They never seem to practise what they preach. 'PSE' was Mr Rogers telling us all about hygiene: washing in one's cracks, changing one's knickers every day (I'm already worried the Y-fronts Mum buys me are making me sterile before I've even had a chance to try), using deodorants, and the evils of nose picking, bum scratching, farting and burping.

Everyone knows what HE's had for breakfast, what brand of fags he smokes, and which beer he drinks for lunch, from his breath at ten yards—it stinks really badly. But he broke his own (and Uncle Bob's) all-time record by farting (the silent 'killer' type), burping, and scratching his bum all at the same time, and then he looked at Sam accusingly.

The polluting smell of stale sweat in the changing room, with unwashed feet in hot pursuit or, as old Will. S. would have it, 'The rankest compound of villainest smell that ever offended nostrils' (The Merry Wives of Windsor), still hangs around in spite of Mr Rogers's talk and his leaflet on 'Keeping It Clean'. It wouldn't make any difference if he went on strike for ever.

Had to write on 'What Makes People Smell' for homework. Supposed to stimulate our interest in the subject. Nearly beheaded myself toppling the library copy of the Oxford Medical Textbook off the shelf. It said (after translation via my medical dictionary) that lots of smells come from special glands called 'aprocrine glands' that are in our armpits, around our nipples (mine are not up to much), and around our prick and bum hole. They don't start working till puberty, and they produce stuff which is a mixture of dead cells and greasy substances. This stuff is all decomposed by bacteria that normally live on the surface of the skin, and this makes chemicals which give us our body odours—the dreaded BO.

In the animal kingdom this smelly stuff is important for marking out territorial areas. Can't imagine anyone marking out our changing room as an important territorial area. Aprocrine glands and their smells are a kind of sexual organ. Wonder why I'm not turned on by Cilla's armpits?

It seems that moths might be, though. There are these things called 'pheromones', which are just small molecules of simple chemical substances floating around in the air like radio waves, giving us messages via our noses. They're like smells, but we don't even notice them, except that they may alter our behaviour. A female moth, the textbook said, could release enough of a chemical called 'bombykol' all at once to attract a trillion males from miles around, in an instant. Luckily she's a bit more restrained and makes do with half a dozen at a time.

What wouldn't I give for a human male equivalent? And there's no saying there isn't one, though it hasn't been discovered yet.

Deodorants work by killing off the bacteria living on the skin. But of course, knocking off all those lovely pheromones at the same time might be cutting short endless subconscious smelly and sexy conversations. Sometimes things you eat, like garlic, come out in these glands; and also changes in the temperature of your body when you're ill increase the rate at which the bacteria work, and make you even more smelly.

Then there's the sweat glands themselves—called 'eccrine glands'—about three to four million of them all over the body, including the hands and face. On a normal day they produce about 500 cubic centimetres of sweat, but they can manage

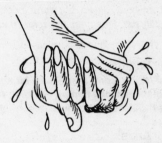

up to three or four litres an hour. Certainly sounds more like 'bathed in sweat' than just 'dripping with'.

It also said that 'man' (somebody should mention sexism and political correctness to these authors) uses the evaporation of sweat from the skin to keep him cool, unlike other animals which use insulation against heat, or panting when they get very hot. Emotion and anxiety also make us sweat. (Telling me—when I finally managed to hold Cilla's hand last week in the cinema, mine must have felt like a wet sponge to her—scares me stiff! Every time she comes near me my brain slips out of gear and I don't know what to say.)

I hate getting sweaty hands and feet, and they don't seem to be the only places—as my underpants keep falling to pieces. Maybe it's because they can't stand the strain of what's inside them. Sally is always going on about how I pong—she doesn't understand that it's all to do with the bacterial breakdown of my skin and clothes.

Got top marks for my PSE. Wouldn't have expected less. Randy Jo had found an article called 'Favourite Words', all about how some doctors had asked a hundred children what their favourite words were for pricks and vaginas. It was wasted on Mr Rogers who said Jo had a dirty mind. Luckily I have a dirty mind, like the doctors who asked the questions, so Jo gave it to me.

Favourite Words for **Penis**:
Willy, cock, *knob*, knob end, *winkle*, penis, *dinkle*, willie warbler, *twinkle*, din-a-ling, *my body*, diggle, *big worm*, prick, *tail*, wotsit, *privates*, winkler, *dilly dat*, little man, *hosepipe*, nudger, *dick*, tinkle, *bum*, Bobbit.

Favourite Words for **Vagina**:
Fanny, vagina, *pinkie*, vag, *cunt*, tweet, *fluffy bit*, tummy, *foo foo*, no willie, *luly*, front bottom, *special tummy*, crumpet, *tuppeny*, ninny, *foo*, cavern, *pocket*, channel tunnel, *wee wee*, twinkle, *private*.

Favourite Words for **Anus**:
Bum, bottom, *arse*, backside, *arse hole*, back passage.

Favourite Words for **Testicles**:
Balls, testicles, *goolies*, privates, *nuts*, rugby balls, *bollocks*.

Favourite Words for **Shitting**:
Poohs, toilet, *loo*, number two, *plops*, sit down, *do a soggy*, dump pooh cheese, *bobs*, big ones, *cack*, plomps, *big toilet*, go bum, *shit*, mud, *kaka*, shite, *popper*, big job.

Favourite Words for **Passing Wind**:
Fart, pardon, *wind*, blow off, *fluffed*, permped, *bum burp*, pop off, *rude noise*, trump, *pass wind*, done one, *cracked a nut*, let polly out, *bottom noise*, whiffed, *bottom spoke*, prout, *guff*, windy pops.

Favourite Words for **Peeing**:
Wee wee, toilet, *loo*, widdle, *bog*, pee pee, *piss*, aunty Jane.

Favourite Words for **Vomiting**:
Sick, puke, *throw up*, chuck, *chunder*, hurl, *barf*, blow chunks.

Pity the guy who calls his prick 'bum'.

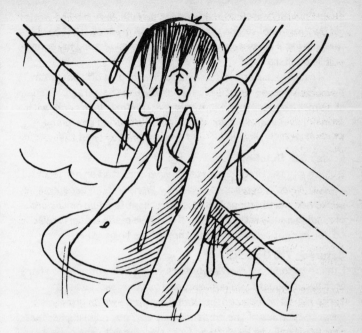

Wednesday 4th October

Got jumped on in the pool today. Nearly drowned. What a way to go—in other people's pee. Mr Rogers was supervising, and as he fished me out he said I should have been more careful as drowning is the third most common cause of death in children, after car accidents and burns, and it is still a lot more likely than me dying of AIDS. I object to this speculation on my future sex life. Anyhow I survived, with stinging eyes—a mixture of pee and chlorine, though I'm not guilty this time. In Mr Rogers's eyes, the pool is a viral and fungal paradise, 'a new hazard at every footstep,' he said with relish.

It's true though. Every time I've caught athletes' foot it's been at the pool, in the changing room, or in the showers. I don't think it's serious, just very agitating. You're trying to get your shoe off to rub the terrible itching between your toes, and hoping nobody will come in and see you. Mum gives me the same old lecture about drying properly between my toes (I'm too old for 'This little piggy went to market') and not wearing my comfy smelly trainers.

I'd rather have smelly feet with skin dropping off than wear black leathers, so I'm still changing shoes in the garage. When the smell gets too bad, Mum subtly stuffs my clean socks with a tin of powder and a tube of cream. I'm a walking pharmacy—Mycil, Daktarin, Myocota—you name them, I've tried them.

Friday 6th October

Susie's got the dreaded warts. They've sprouted on her thumb. I think they look horrendous and dirty. Wonder if it's because she sucks her thumb? Hope I don't catch them. It would be the end of holding hands with Cilla—just when I've made a start. I want to ask her out again but don't know where to take her.

Saturday 7th October

Susie's becoming a real toady wart-hog. She's got them on her feet too. I thought you got verrucas on your feet, but that turns out to be just another name for warts which grow inwards because of the pressure. Susie's busy painting her feet with stuff called salicylic acid from the chemist. She says it kills off the warty skin and then YOU have to scrape the dead skin off.

Don't much like having a bath after her—not that I have one very often. At least now she's got something other than her weight to worry about.

Sunday 8th October

Three of Susie's friends came to 'play'. Tea consisted of wart talk. Put me right off my egg and toast.

Her friend Kate said you had to get hold of a piece of raw steak, rub it on the wart, and bury it. Trouble was when she did it her dog kept digging it up and eating it. Her mum said to use Pedigree Chum next time, as it was cheaper, and anyhow her wart had spread. Now she was trying her gran's recipe—wiping it with the juice of a dandelion stalk, and putting the broken dandelion on to the thorn of a rose bush. With luck, when it died her wart would fall off. If it didn't her gran's next best remedy was attending three funerals, and saying each time, as the funeral bells were ringing, 'Please take my warts with you.'

Mum said that when she was young (a long time ago) you had to spit on your warty hands every morning. She tried it and it didn't work, but then she kept forgetting.

Mary said Susie could try peeing on her hands, but I suggested the local swimming pool instead.

Monday 9th October
Worried. Something's growing on my knee. No one's hand has been there recently, but I'm spitting on it every hour, just in case. Keep missing but it helps clean my shoes.

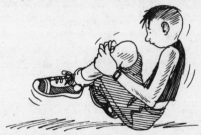

Friday 13th October
Mum's taking Susie to someone called 'a podiatrist' tomorrow to have her verrucas fixed. Didn't explain to Mum about my knee, but said I would come too, to keep them company.

Saturday 14th October
A podiatrist turns out to be a 'foot specialist'—smelly work if my feet are anything to go by. She said the spot on my knee wasn't a wart, just a pimple, and it would be better if I stopped spitting on it. She checked my feet, and gave me a lecture on how important it is to have well-fitting shoes. Otherwise you can get corns and callouses which are caused by rubbing from badly-fitting shoes. They are not something you catch, which is what I had thought.

When it came to Susie's feet (and I don't know how she could stand getting close to THEM), she got quite excited and started a new lecture about how warts, whether on the hands or the feet, ARE catching. They happen when wart viruses (and apparently there are several different kinds) get into cracks or cuts in the skin. As with my athletes' foot, swimming baths and changing rooms are common places to get the infections. They happen most in children aged 12 to 16, but some children NEVER get them, some get just the odd one, and some get lots and lots. No one knows why (there seems to be a lot that people don't know about when it comes down to it).

Over half of the warts disappear in two years, even if you do nothing about them. Probably explains why all that digging meat into the ground, and going to funerals, SEEMS to work. If you use any of the medical treatments, like salicylic acid, then three-quarters will clear up in three months, which seems a bit better. For the ones that don't go away with this treatment, then burning, freezing or scraping away the dead skin often helps.

All this seemed to make Susie feel happier, though she had expected hers to go away overnight after she had tried the acid, and she didn't fancy the burning or freezing parts. The foot doc said Susie can go swimming as long as she wears a plaster to cover her verrucas.

Sunday 15th October

Bits of Susie's dead skin on the bathroom floor this morning. Used downstairs bog instead.

Sam came round reeking of so much Lynx that it was difficult to breathe. Told him that although in the natural world there are lovely smells, like flowers, it doesn't mean that they suit humans.

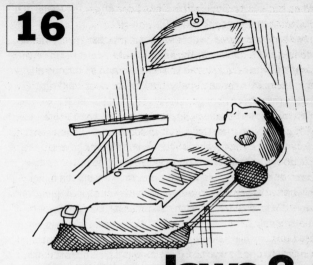

16

And so to Jaws 3

Tuesday 24th October

Randy Jo took Cilla to the cinema again last night. Spent all his time telling me about it today. I hate him. His acne's even worse than mine and he spends his pocket money on *Playboy*. I'm surprised he'd want to take Cilla out after spending all his nights with Miss October. Anyhow, last time I got near her at the cinema, I thought her breath smelt a bit—not enough to put me off though. Maybe she thinks I smell? I'll borrow Sam's Lynx.

Read this thing in the *Guinness Book of Records* about someone in Minnesota, USA, called Alfred Wolson, who kissed 8,000 people in 8 hours on 15 September 1990, which is 1 person every 3.6 seconds.

Wednesday 25th October

Mum took us both to the new dentist. She said we were lucky to find one who still worked for the National Health Service, and would give us our treatment free if we were under 18. These are now rarer than hen's teeth.

Just because Susie had a final fitting for her brace, Mum suddenly had to remember me as well. I was scared stiff of the old dentist, who would pin me to the chair and be furious if I as much as screamed occasionally. Luckily she went bankrupt. Serves her right.

Hate dentists because they're bigger liars than politicians. They say they won't hurt you, but you come out in agony, with lips feeling the size of a blue baboon's bum. Some have traces of being human—like this new one. He's nice—has outer space gadgets and makes jokes all the time. With my mouth full of bits of metal it's easier to laugh than answer stupid questions. He says it's boring dealing with rotten teeth every day, just because people can't be bothered to clean them. He gave me a leaflet to read while he was poking around in Susie's mouth. Took an extra one to give to Cilla. I know it'll piss her off but I don't care. Anybody who goes out with Randy Jo has to be a slag.

GOOD TEETH, GOOD LOOKS

Good teeth, bad teeth, it's not chance

Remember, neglect your teeth and they soon start to look dingy. Worse still they can decay and cause pain. And they can also create an unpleasant smell and taste in your mouth.

This leaflet will help you get to know what's good for your teeth and what's bad for them. You should ask your dentist for any further advice and practical assistance you need.

Despite what you may have heard, it's not chance that will help you keep your teeth and your looks. It's knowing what to do and then doing it.

ENEMIES

'Tooth Decay' ✗

What happens is that sugar and bacteria in the mouth get together and make an acid. This acid attacks the tooth enamel first, and then deeper. And that can hurt! To your teeth, sugar is enemy No. 1.

Sugar ✗

You don't need it. Your teeth hate it. And it is worst if you're forever munching sweet things and having fizzy drinks between meals. That's how most damage is done. If you do like your sweets and cola, cut them down to just after meals.

'Plaque' ✗

We've all got it. Run your tongue round your teeth and you'll feel a furry, glue-like substance. That's 'plaque'. But don't worry. It's how long plaque stays at any one time and is allowed to build up that matters. That's why brushing is so important. The bacteria in plaque cause gum disease—the earliest sign of this is that your gums bleed when they are brushed. In the end, the gum and bone supporting the teeth may be destroyed, causing the teeth to become loose and to fall out.

Bleeding gums ✗

There's nothing natural about your gums bleeding—even if they don't hurt. And if you don't brush your teeth often enough, you may start seeing blood on your toothbrush. Should this happen, then (surprisingly perhaps!) you really should start brushing your teeth more frequently. And if that doesn't put things right, see your dentist.

FRIENDS

Your toothbrush, naturally ✓

Almost certainly you already brush your teeth, but do you do it properly? It isn't easy. The difficult part is to remove plaque where the gums meet the teeth. Your dentist will show you exactly where to brush and how to do it.

Regular brushing is important too. You do your hair every day— why not do your teeth every day?

Fluoride ✓

Use a fluoride toothpaste. Fluoride is a naturally occurring substance which is present in small quantities in many foods—such as tea or fish—as well as in water. It unites with tooth enamel and makes teeth stronger, less likely to decay. But most of us don't get enough of it from natural sources so we need it in toothpaste.

Try something tasty and safe between meals ✓

Why sweets anyway? Try nuts, fruit, carrots or celery. Look around and you'll find many enjoyable tasty bites that won't harm your teeth.

THE DENTIST

A friend indeed!

Don't for a minute think that your dentist is there only to drill, fill or extract. In fact, regular visits could mean he or she never has to do those things for you! Your dentist will check your teeth carefully and care for them when necessary and give you all the advice you need about looking after them between visits.

Look upon your dentist as someone who will help you KEEP your teeth. And your looks.

What a patronizing git!

I had to have a filling, and the worst bit was when he crammed cotton wool pads, a sucker thing, and a drill into my mouth at the same time. Thought I was going to drown in my own spit and spent most of the time trying not to swallow.

While all this was happening he burbled on about how all that your teeth need is ONE really good thorough brush every day, with any toothbrush and (most important) with FLUORIDATED toothpaste. If everybody did this, or the government fluoridated all drinking water, like they do in Moscow, New York, Birmingham, Dublin and Sydney; and if people gave up eating sweets and other sugary things all the time, and just ate them occasionally, say on Wednesdays and Saturdays, then teeth problems would almost disappear. But the average English schoolchild eats 118 grams of sugar EVERY day. Sugar is converted into acid by bacteria in the mouth and starts eating into the enamel of the teeth within a few seconds.

He went on about how many old people have NO teeth of their own—not one! (Gran's like this. She keeps all her spare false teeth in a plastic bag in her bathroom cupboard.) About half of children aged 15 have had at least ONE filling (I'm now part of this statistic). He then gave me a lecture about tooth brushing, using thorough, small backwards and forwards scrubbing movements, gently all over all the teeth, inside and out, and particularly where the tooth goes into the gum. Didn't sound difficult as I do it already.

At least I'm not 'brace faced' like Susie, who's got to wear this cage at night—'for your own good', as Mum said—because the front teeth on her top jaw are crooked and stick out, and there is a big gap between them (like the bride of Dracula) which she can't clean with a normal toothbrush.

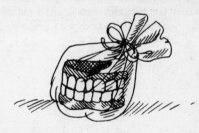

Friday 27th October
Sssusie sssays that it'sss like having ssseventeen sssets of teeth. Ssshe ssspeaks like thisss all the time.

Saturday 28th October
Susie's nagging Mum for compensation over her brace. She wants her ears pierced. Two of her friends at school have just done each other's—with a needle which they tried to 'sterilize' by holding it over a candle. Mum was HORRIFIED. She said you can get all sorts of infections that way—like AIDS and

hepatitis. She said she'd had hers done when she was 20, but if Susie really wanted hers done now she must go somewhere licensed where they'd use proper sterilized packs.

I suppose Mum should be grateful that it's only her ears Susie wants done, as nipple piercing is all the rage in America—though I don't think they would find anything on Susie to pierce. I'll ask Cilla what she thinks. It sounds fantastically painful. I think Randy Jo should have his ego extension pierced. That would be even more painful, which would serve him right.

Sal, as usual, is a real expert. She has five in one ear alone and a nose ring. But she agrees it's best to have them done properly in a shop, even if it does cost a bit more. She had hers done at different times, and the best one was when her current boyfriend gave her nine-carat gold sleepers to put in. The cheap sleepers she had used before had always made her ears all pussy. Sal said last time she went, the woman had pointed out that the actual piercing was only the beginning. It was really important to keep the sleepers in for a whole month, to keep the ear lobes very clean, and to turn the sleepers regularly.

None of this seems to have put Susie off. She's having them done next week.

17

Days off School

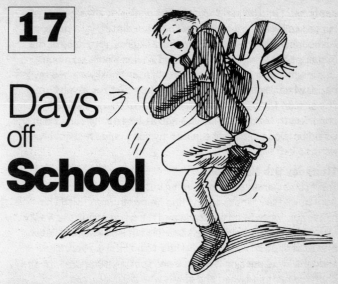

Monday 6th November

Our street firework party was ruined. I sometimes think it's a pity Guy Fawkes didn't manage to blow up the Houses of Parliament and himself too.

Nick DID get blown up last night—both by a rocket and by his parents: and his parents got blown up by the local GP on call when they took him to have the burns on his face treated. He had to go to hospital, where they said he'd got 'second degree burns', which means blisters, red streaking and oozing of the skin, with a lot of pain. They put this special non-stick dressing on and said he might need a skin graft. He would probably be scarred for life, and was lucky not to have been blinded.

MY only mistake was to pick up a used sparkler before it had cooled down. Luckily Mum had just been reading my first-aid book which said to put my hand into cold water IMMEDIATELY (not ice) and leave it there for AT LEAST five minutes. This cooled the burn, stopped too many cells from getting

destroyed, and helped the pain. The book also stressed that
burns like Nick's had to be treated immediately by a doctor.
Although to begin with my burn hurt like hell, very deep burns
apparently damage the nerves and so don't hurt so much.

This morning I had a great long blister (luckily across my left
hand) which I want to pop, but Mum won't let me as she says
the skin on the blister is protecting the damaged cells
underneath from infection. It's not as bad as my sunburn in the
summer though. It throbs inside my head, and I feel wobbly, so
went to bed early.

Thursday 9th November

Tried to get dressed this morning but gave up. Curled up on the
sofa downstairs instead and had just got comfy, with the
heater on, when Mum walked in and flared up about the waste
of electricity. I explained I felt terrible but she wouldn't listen,
and said that if I was really ill I had to go back to bed. She
thought I was putting it on, but she took my temperature and
changed her mind when she saw it was 39.5 degrees
centigrade. It's funny. Although it was up 2.5 degrees, I actually
felt shivery. I wonder how high one's temperature can go? I bet
one would die after about 45 degrees . . . feel as if I'm on my way
there.

Mum rang the doctor and she came to see me. Said it was
probably JUST 'flu and caused by a virus. It will be better in
three or four days, and there is no treatment except to stay in
bed if I feel like it, have lots of clear drinks, and take
paracetamol every four to six hours. The paracetamol will bring
my temperature down and help my headache. If I die it'll be all
her fault.

I told her about the headaches I've been having, like the one I
had when Mum and Dad were having their 'discussions'. She
looked in the back of my eyes with a light—like they did at the
hospital when I had my accident. She told me it wasn't a brain
tumour or meningitis, or anything else seriously wrong, which
I'm glad about, as I had been worrying. She said if it was
meningitis it would hurt to bend my neck and I'd be much iller.

She was a bit nosy about my life at school and at home, but said there are lots of causes for headaches, like being a bit tense, or not being very well, but usually they go away without you knowing what caused them. If it is migraine, she said, the headache will often be on one side, and you get funny lines across your eyesight before the headache starts. It runs in families, but no one in MY family has it, thank goodness.

She also said that if ever I was worried about things, I could come and talk to her. I didn't have to bring Mum or Dad along, and she would treat anything that I said as 'confidential'. I didn't understand what 'confidential' meant, so she explained that if I didn't want her to, she wouldn't tell anything I said to anyone else, including my parents. Sounds OK to me.

After she left, I went from being shivery to being soaked in sweat. You could have fried an egg on me. I flung all my bedclothes off, and told Mum I wanted to go easy on the paracetamol because I had read somewhere that having a bit of a temperature may help to kill off the infection. I took one though, just to help my throbbing headache. Can't write any more. It hurts too much.

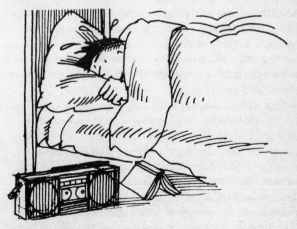

Friday 10th November

Dying, though did manage a few games of Nintendo. Nobody cares. They'll be sorry when it's too late, except for Mum, who's the best nurse anyone could have. My thermometer says 40 degrees.

Saturday 11th November

Didn't die after all. Temperature down to 38.5. Susie's in a flap because one of her pierced ears has gone pussy. Mum says to keep bathing it with the lotion they gave her and it will soon clear up.

Randy Jo's had his nose pierced! Somewhat less painful than the latest place I had in mind for him, alas. Why hasn't Cilla rung me up to find out if I'm dead?

Monday 13th November

Temperature 37.0 degrees—normal again. Susie's not well now. She came home early, not the 'flu (yet!). She wouldn't tell me what was wrong, but after a bit of third degree admitted it was period pains. I know she's started 'officially' now.

I'm feeling better today, but at first it was horrible. I felt so ill. My head felt as if it was going to burst. I couldn't sleep, and the nights went so slowly it was just a matter of waiting for morning. I ached and I was hot, but my joints were freezing. Mum's very grumpy about us being at home, maybe because she can't go to work, but I've diagnosed the 'flu and told her to take paracetamol and go to bed.

Spent part of the day watching baby programmes, *Neighbours* (Helen Daniels is as annoying as Mum, with all her 'good' advice), gratuitous violence, and a programme on the human brain. My headache's gone. I learnt that Turgenev, a Russian writer, had the heaviest brain ever recorded. They cut him up and weighed it in at 2,012 grams, whereas an average man's brain weighs 1,410 grams. I also spent some time writing and reading books in my room. In fact, I stuffed my superbrain (which is ten times the size of a gorilla's, even though the hairy beast weighs three or four times more than my mum) with facts about my body.

It holds 5 litres of blood, and my heart pumps 90 cubic centimetres at every beat; so normally about 5 litres, or the complete amount of blood in my body, every minute. This can go up to 30 litres (all my blood being pumped around my body 6 times in a minute) during hard exercise.

Other facts about my heart are: it weighs about 260 grams and the most normal rate it beats at is 70–75 beats a minute. But it can go very rapidly from 45 beats per minute when resting to 200 beats during exercise. The heart is made up of 200,000,000,000 cells, which certainly seems amazing when you think that the whole body starts off as just two.

There are 96,560 kilometres of arteries, veins, and blood capillaries in the human body, through which all this blood travels. I also learnt from TV that there are 1,000,000,000,000 nerve cells in our brain. And after we are 18 we lose a thousand of these every day. (I wonder whose job it is counting all these cells and measuring how long all the blood vessels are?) Our kidneys filter 90 litres of blood per day, which means that all the blood in our body is filtered 17 times every 24 hours, but only about 2 litres of waste a day comes out as pee.

Susie keeps barging into my room to see what I'm doing. Wish she would knock. It could be really embarrassing. She's bored. I told her to buzz off, till she told me I'd missed another sex talk at school. She knows my weak spots all right. Sudden change of interest on my part. Luckily she'd brought home a leaflet.

YOU CAN SAY 'NO!'

Your body belongs to *you*

Sometimes you can know someone for a long time and like them a lot and then they'll start to do things you don't like at all. Perhaps they'll start touching you in a way that seems strange to you, but since you like the person and he's always been nice to you, you don't like to ask him to stop. But you can and you should. Because you don't have to let anyone touch you in a way you don't like, even if it's an adult you've always got on well with. Or even if it's someone in your own family. Or a neighbour.

Strangers

You've probably been told many times not to take sweets from strangers, or get into a car with someone you don't know, because they might do bad things to you. But people we know well can also do bad things to us, by making us believe they are *not* bad.

It's not special to be sexually abused!

A person might tell you that what he feels about you is something very special, and that you must keep it secret because other people would not understand. And perhaps he makes *you* feel very special. However, this happens to many girls and boys, and it is *not* special.

It's unfair if a grown-up makes you do things you don't understand

In fact, the grown-up (or sometimes it's a teenager) is being very unfair, because he is bigger than you and knows more about everything. So he can easily get you to do things you don't really want to. So that later on, when you *do* understand, you'll feel very angry. I'm saying 'he' all the time, but it can sometimes be a woman.

Find someone who can help you

If you can't get the person to stop bothering you and you can't keep out of his way, you should tell someone you think will help you—a schoolteacher, or your mother, or an older sister, or a policewoman, for instance. If you tell one person and they don't believe you, or are too frightened to help you, then try someone else, and keep trying till you find someone who *will* help you.

Also, tell your friends, so that they can stay away from that person too, and their parents can help.

Don't be bullied

And if one of your friends tells you about someone bothering her, then try to help her in every way you can, because it's horrible to be alone with a problem like this. You start thinking things, like 'There must be something wrong with me or he wouldn't have done that.' But in fact there's nothing wrong with you at all. You're not the problem. *He* is.

You are not to blame

It *is* frightening when something like this happens, but you can be sure it's all right to say 'No!' and you can be sure, too, that it's not your fault. It's nothing *you've* done which made this person behave in the way he did. He has probably done it to other children, and he will certainly go on doing it if he is not stopped. We don't like telling tales, but this is different. If you tell people, he can be stopped.

REMEMBER, IT'S YOUR BODY AND YOU CAN SAY 'NO!'

Susie said she reckoned that the talk was because of what happened to one of her friends. Practically nobody but Susie knows, but about a week ago, when Jane was on her way home, a car stopped and a man she knew as a friend of her parents asked her the way to the local superstore. He pretended he didn't understand her directions and said could she just hop in and guide him. Susie said Jane had always been a real dumbo— the type that would be kind to King Kong if she met him in the street—and she got in. He started putting his hand up her skirt, and saying dirty things about touching his prick. Jane got very angry and began screaming, so he became all friendly and nice again, and tried to bribe her with sweets not to say anything. He said it had to be THEIR special secret, and that they would both get into terrible trouble if anyone found out.

Jane didn't know what to do because she thought her mum would be furious, but she told her all the same. Her mum said it wasn't Jane's fault, it was all the man's, which made her feel much better. A couple of days later, when Jane was less upset, her mum said that the man was having special treatment, and was going to move far away to another town.

Susie said the sex talk at school was just what Mum and Dad had said a million times about not accepting lifts or presents of any kind from strangers, and even perhaps being a bit careful of friends! It is sometimes really difficult to tell the difference between when people are just being nice to one another, and hugging or kissing, and when somebody is trying to do something nasty to you. Mum says the best thing is being aware that it might happen. And if it does, saying 'NO' and meaning it, and saying it with one's whole body—pushing away, getting angry (instead of being frozen with fear), and ALWAYS telling someone. Best of all is not getting into situations that you don't know how to get out of, though some things, like flashers in churches and other pervs, are difficult to avoid.

Susie said she is going to learn self-defence. I can't exactly see her chopping someone in half at a single blow, but I said I think it's a good idea. Women of the family ALL into period problems. Silence falls as Dad or me approach. Told Dad I'd try and find us an all-male problem—but could only come up with CDS, which is much more frequent than the monthlies and stands for Cilla Deprivation Syndrome.

Tuesday 14th November

Feel mixed about going back to school. Getting really bored being at home, but I'll have loads of work to catch up with when I get back. Bet no one believes I've been ill. None of my mates have been to see me.

Wednesday 15th November

Good to see my friends again, but now Sam's away with the 'flu. Seems it's going round the whole school. We had to have a supply teacher for games, as Mr Jones has it too. Hope the supply teacher gets something worse. He said he thought I was skiving when I said I felt too tired to play football.

Thursday 16th November

Borrowed this really funny book, called Man's Best Friend, all about willies with a life of their own. Might lend it to Cilla. I'm back on her again.

Tests in maths and biology next week. I was worried that I might have missed some stuff for them while I was ill, but luckily the first thing we got taught in maths today was about revising and how not to get stressed. Last year, when I was doing tests on the human body, I didn't know where to start. I thought I had to learn the name of every bone in the body. Another problem is that I never feel I have time to do all the questions.

What I'm doing is looking at everything I'm meant to cover, sorting it out into different topics, and making a timetable so that I cover everything, sketchily at least, in the time I've got, instead of getting hung up on doing one thing really thoroughly.

Another thing they said is that we can only concentrate for so long, so it is best to work for an hour and then have a break—watch telly, play a game on Super Nintendo, or whatever.

Wednesday 22nd November
Worried—I hate tests.

Thursday 23rd November
Wiped out. Two tests today. Completely forgot in the first one what the teachers said about timing. I only completed fourteen out of twenty questions in the maths, as I got stuck on the third one and wasted lots of time. It didn't help finding out that Sam found the last six questions really easy.
I did better in biology. There were ten questions to do in two hours. First I read them all carefully for ten minutes so that I understood what they were about, and then I really concentrated on answering each question for ten minutes only. That left ten minutes at the end for my nightmare spelling.

18 Four **EYES**

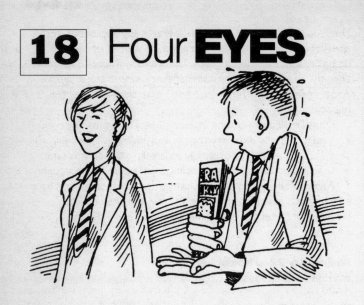

Monday 27th November

Another bad day. Mrs Smellie moved me to the front of the class for 'not concentrating'. Was concentrating, but on copying out Sam's homework on a topic that I'd missed when I had 'flu. Was made to abandon my desk at the back, specially chosen to be out of the teacher's view. So furious and embarrassed, I stomped to the front, clutching my things. Dropped latest copy of *Practical Photography* as I passed Cilla and because it was something I'd looked at rather a lot, it fell open at a page revealing a woman who was completely starkers. I blushed to the roots of my acned hair follicles (though these have improved recently), and insisted to the class that the magazine had been bought for photographic purposes only. As I got myself sorted out, I swear I heard Cilla mutter, 'Me thinks he doth protest too much.'

When I'd stopped sulking, I noticed that I could ACTUALLY READ what was on the board without screwing up my eyes or copying off my neighbour. This may improve my work, but am I going blind?

Tuesday 28th November

Another puncture. Found I'd left the top off the tube of rubber solution, which had dried up. Unsuccessfully tried to blame Susie. Took bus to school and nearly got on the wrong one, as I could only see the number when it was very close. Even more worried about going blind. Will I have to wear glasses, like Dad? Can't stand even thinking about it—too grim.

Wednesday 29th November

Came top in biology. Told Cilla it was all the practical experience I had had that had helped. My maths I am not revealing. Raj came top. Some of the brainiest and hardest people in our class are either Asian or West Indian.

In trouble at home. Bent all the teaspoons trying to lever off my tyre. Susie turned out to be an expert at puncture mending and said she'd do it when she got back from her self-defence class. Tried offering her 10p per puncture for the future, but she successfully negotiated 20p. Bet she becomes a union boss when she grows up, and growing up she certainly seems to be.

Looked in the mirror to try and imagine what I would look like with pebbles on. At least they might hide some of the zits.

Monday 4th December

Got a note today for Mum about an eye test at school next week. Apparently they do one every two or three years. First note I haven't left in my pocket to dissolve in the washing machine (Mum loves me for this). Bit worried about the eye test in case I fail and need glasses, especially as on the way home Sam called John 'Four Eyes'. John said, 'Four eyes are better than two,' and when someone else said, 'What's it like walking around with double glazing?' all he said was, 'I have the best—Everest!' Doesn't seem to worry him, but I kept unusually quiet.

Monday 11th December

The day of the TEST. Kept trying to see if I could read the bus numbers on the way to school, but no, they were just a blur in the distance through the drizzle. Luck however was on my side, as the eye test was done during my PE lesson. Unlike at lunch-time, everyone was trying to get to the BACK of the queue, so as to miss as much school as possible. The school nurse, Hazel Chops, who looks ancient and must have had at least eighteen children (perhaps that's why they chose her?) turned a cold eye on us all, which silenced us like a laser beam.

My turn came at last. I stood in front of the chart, which they seemed to have put about five miles away, and could only read to the third line before the letters blurred out. Felt really panicky, like when I know I am going to fail an exam. Tried to remember the letters from the last time I had had the test, but couldn't. Asked old Guzzler Guts Gary (whose breath not only kills at forty metres, but who will do almost anything for a bribe of a sweet—hence the rotten teeth and pongo breath) to read the letters on the chart and whisper them to me. Alas, even HIS greed grew dim under the school nurse's gaze. What a lightweight. I failed and failed miserably.

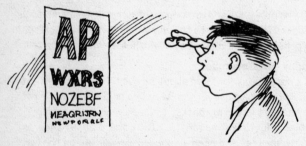

Hazel Chops turned out to be nice, even if she was a bit crinkly. When she realized how unhappy I was, she pointed out it wasn't a question of 'failing' but of not being able to see. She also said not to worry, she was sure there was nothing seriously wrong but that I should go and see an optician who would test my eyes more thoroughly. I told her I hated the idea of wearing glasses, then I noticed that she was wearing them which made me feel dead embarrassed. She explained that at my age, about one in five children wear glasses, and by her age nearly everyone does (96 per cent was how she put it). So there is no harm in getting used to them early. This made me feel a bit better but I still don't go for the idea.

At least I passed the colour test, where they make you read a whole lot of numbers made up of different coloured dots. This is to see if you can tell the difference between green and red colours, and if you fail you can't become an airline pilot or an electrician. Not that I want to be either, because I actually want to be a famous scientist and most of them wear specs anyway.

Think I'll give up telly in case Mum's right and it's too much watching which has strained my eyes.

Thursday 14th December

Went with Sam and some friends to see a '15' film—my first try at getting in so was terrified, even though my birthday's on Sunday. We'd fixed to buy a ticket for John, because although he's the oldest of us all—16 next month—his eyes hardly come up to the level of the kiosk, which we thought might cause problems! All went fine till the wimp checking the tickets on the way in asked John if he was standing in a hole or something, and said if not, then he wasn't going in. So we all stayed out in sympathy, which depleted my daily quota of visual sex.

Needless to say, it made John furious as a teacher at school had already asked him that day what the weather was like 'down there'. I knew how he felt, as I am sure I'm going to get teased about the specs. Told him about growth hormone treatment but it turns out he's already had all the tests.

Saturday 16th December

Trip to the optician—a shop in the High Street that I had cycled past every day without noticing. One can be blind in more ways than one.

The optician made me sit in a chair in a dark room filled with funny lights and gadgets. I told her which lines in something looking like a cart wheel were clearest; and read from all sorts of different charts while she popped pieces of glass into frames in front of my eyes (like pennies going into a slot machine). She smelt nice (unlike many I could name). Then she took a close look into my eyes with a light she called an 'opthalmoscope', the same as the doctor used in the hospital when I had my accident and at home when I had my headaches. (I had to look it up in the dictionary for the spelling.)

After lots of tests, it turned out I have short sight and will need glasses, which is now no surprise. The optician helped by saying that each of us is made slightly different from everyone else (thank goodness for that). But just as some people are short and some are tall, so some are born with eyeballs one shape and some with them another. (I wonder how far these differences go?) She said that it is not that eyes are 'bad' or 'good', but that everyone sees more or less clearly and if you already see fairly clearly then you don't need glasses, but the less clearly you see, the more you do need them.

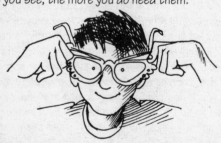

There are two main reasons for needing glasses. SHORT SIGHTED, which is what I am, means that things far away look blurred, but things close to look clear (when reading, for instance, or looking at *Practical Photography*). LONG SIGHTED is when you can see things far away quite clearly (like the numbers on the bus, long before it reaches you), but can't see clearly the words in a book or newspaper.

I can go back to watching TV, as there is no evidence that this or reading in poor light strains the eyes. (Reading in poor light just makes it difficult to read.) The optician also told me that most headaches have nothing to do with eyesight.

I then had to choose some frames, as I wanted some that made me look clever but not an actual boff. It seems stupid having a whole lot of boring-looking glasses. This isn't going to help to encourage people to wear them. The optician said I needed two pairs, because I was bound to break or lose one sometime. I bet Mum £5 I wouldn't lose mine. Might put the money towards saving for contact lenses.

Sunday 17th December
Cilla left my bi.thday supper with Randy Jo. Totally wrecked today. He's always on the pull. Sam said she was only going out with him because she felt sorry for him—but what about me?

Wednesday 20th December
What a way to spend the first morning of the holidays. No lie-in till midday, and cooking myself an egg or two, with bacon and fried toast, after everybody else has gone out. This morning it was up at nine, for a last glance at my face without pebbles. My moustache has gone. I borrowed Dad's electric shaver. He doesn't know, but I hope he gives me one for Christmas, all the same. Now I'm off to the optician's. Won't wear my glasses on the way home, in case anyone I know sees me.

Thursday 21st December
Wore glasses inside the house only. Susie said they looked good in such a sarcastic way it was impossible to believe her. Mum and Dad were encouraging though, especially Dad who now has a 'glasses ally' in the family. Noticed a red mark around the top of my nose where the glasses sit, something else to ruin my appearance. Dad said it often happens like that when you first get specs, but gradually the skin gets used to them.

Saturday 23rd December
Met Cilla Christmas shopping in town. She liked my glasses—and me, for once. She even asked me to party tonight at her cousin's. Is she just asking me because she feels sorry for me? Not sure I want to go after what happened at the last party we were at together.

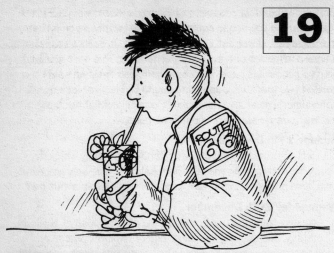

Drunken Desires

Monday 25th December

Tore the last two pages out. It's evening on Christmas Day. What I'd written before was too confused (like me), so I'm starting again, to try and sort things out. I'm all churned up and can't cope. It's to do with Cilla, and me, and parties, and what to do next, or whether to do anything, all mixed up with me supposed to be feeling good because it's Christmas. That's in fact what started the whole problem off.

The reason I hadn't wanted to go to the party with Cilla was because the last party I had been to was pretty boring. This was partly because everybody was drinking and I wasn't, partly because some gatecrashers came and ruined it, and partly because everyone else had a girlfriend. But this time Cilla was asking me. Mum said that I ought to go as I couldn't be unsociable all my life.

It was the first time I'd been to a party knowing only one

person. Till now, I've only been to parties with lots of people the same age as me, like all my friends at school, so on the whole they've been friendly and unthreatening. This one was different. Cilla's cousin is 18, so Cilla and I were the youngest by far, and personally I felt that I was totally different from everyone else and didn't fit in. But Cilla seemed to know everybody, and immediately went off leaving me in total isolation.

The party was in this huge room, and I had to walk across it to a table, around which most of these strangers were sitting. At first I felt very self-conscious because I thought they were all staring at me, but I soon realized they were in fact totally ignoring me. I began to panic inside, when to my relief Cilla suddenly appeared and offered me a drink. I just took what she offered me and drank it down, almost without noticing what it was, I was so nervous and so anxious to seem hard. No one spoke to me, and I couldn't think of anything to say to them. Someone filled up my glass from a bottle on the table, and to cover my embarrassment, and give me something to do, I kept taking nervous sips of wine.

Then someone offered me some Pimm's No. 1, which I'd never had before. I gulped that down too. After a while, the combination of the wine and the music made me feel a bit more relaxed, and I started talking to someone who knew some people I knew. It was only when I got up to go and pee that I realized how drunk I was. I knew that I shouldn't drink any more even if it did relax me and make me able to talk. Suddenly I seemed to lose my shyness entirely and I began to laugh hysterically at something someone said. Cilla came over looking very annoyed and tried to shut me up, but I just made things worse by talking a whole lot of rubbish to her.

As I talked I began to collapse and feel incredibly ill. I sat down, and then almost lay down, with my head between my knees, feeling all cold, sweaty and horrible. I thought I must be dying, I felt so ill. I was convinced Cilla would disappear in embarrassment, but actually she was great, and said that she'd ring my dad, and come back with me.

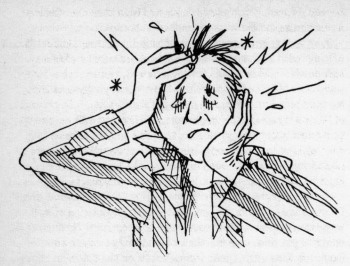

I threw up in the car on the way home. Luckily Cilla was sitting in the front. Mum made me drink lots of water, muttering something about 'preventing dehydration', and put me to bed. She was obviously absolutely spare, but didn't say anything. I don't remember too much after that.

On Christmas Eve I stayed in bed till lunch-time. I was knackered, I had a splitting headache, and my mouth felt as if someone had shat in it. My first hangover. I could have done without Susie smirking and teasing me about getting drunk and liking Cilla. I doubted whether Cilla liked me. Even I didn't like me after last night. I remembered what a fool I'd made of myself, and knew it was going to ruin Christmas.

Mum and Dad haven't said much about it, there's just an uncomfortable feeling around the house. Wish they'd say SOMETHING. I hung up my stocking, and heard Dad come in at 2 a.m., stumbling around and leaving a whisky smell behind him.

Today Susie and Sally came in to open their stockings with me. You'd think Sally was past stockings, but I think she wants to believe in Father Christmas even more than we do. Mum cooked an ace lunch. Noticed Susie had forgotten about being a vegetarian. Turkeys must count as chickens.

Subtle Dad gave Susie a drop of wine but not me. He said I'd had enough. I think I must have gone red, because Susie gave me one of her smug smiles. It provoked Sally though (who last year had done a special topic on alcohol) into announcing that nine out of ten children had tasted an alcoholic drink by the age of 14, and that most of these had tried alcohol at home, closely controlled by their parents. At this, Susie took a 'closely controlled' gulp, spat it out, and said it was disgusting and she couldn't understand how people drank wine. I wondered how much of Sally's topic was done from personal experience! All this talk of alcohol made me feel sick again, so Sally stopped. She said she'd lend me what she'd written, if I was interested.

Brilliant presents from Mum and Dad—a new Walkman and some tapes. Sally gave me soap, Susie a handkerchief, and the much-needed electric razor came from terrible Uncle Bob.

Tuesday 26th December
Boxing Day. Everyone else seems silent and a bit hungover. No sympathy from me. Played my new tapes. Bored by evening. Read Sally's 'Topic on Alcohol' so I could explain the dangers to my family.

TOPIC ON ALCOHOL by Sally Payne
Form VI Lower

Introduction
Alcohol is a chemical whose formula is C_2H_5OH. It is both a poison and a drug and was around long before Christ was born.

Wonder if Jesus ever got drunk? He seemed to do a lot of turning water into wine.

It's made by fermentation and can be produced from all kinds of things like potatoes, flowers, berries, etc., but the common alcoholic drinks are wine which is made from grapes, *cider from apples, beer from hops and barley, gin from barley, malt or rye, flavoured with juniper berries. Rice makes sake, which is Japan's national drink.*

A liquid containing just less than 50 per cent of alcohol by weight is called 'proof spirit'. This is because it contains the smallest amount of alcohol which, when gunpowder is soaked in it, would burn. At least one billion gallons of proof spirit are produced each year and mostly used for drinking. A small amount of alcohol will make people more lively, but larger amounts dull their senses and their brains and they may become unconscious or even die if they take too much.

Perhaps I could make a fortune distilling but I'd certainly remain a teetotaller myself.

Pure alcohol is called 'absolute' alcohol and is very difficult to make. The spirit used in industry and for cleaning paint brushes and things in the home is a mixture of ethyl and methyl alcohol. It is extremely dangerous to drink because the methyl alcohol is so poisonous. Sometimes people have added this to drinks as a joke and other people have been poisoned or blinded, and have even died.

Felt as if someone did that to my drinks at the party before Christmas.

<u>Facts about Alcoholic Drinks</u>
It's how much pure alcohol there is in a drink that is important, but additives which give drinks their colour, flavour, smell and taste also affect how bad the hangover is. Half a pint of beer or lager = one measure (140 millilitres) of spirits (whisky, gin, vodka, etc.) = a glass of wine = a small glass of sherry = a bit less than half a pint of cider.

Hadn't realized that cider's even stronger than beer. Must be careful how much I drink. I always thought it was weaker, and just tossed it back.

Alcohol is rapidly absorbed from the stomach into the blood stream; most is burnt up in the liver and the rest is got rid of in sweat and urine. It is more rapidly absorbed on an empty stomach than a full one, and therefore it's better to eat before you drink. In general it takes the body one hour to get rid of one standard drink. More than five drinks at a party and you won't feel all right again till next morning. Drinking two and a half pints of beer or cider, or the equivalent, in an hour puts you over the legal limit for driving.

The Dangers
In the short term, the main danger is that alcohol affects your judgement, self-control and skills. Road accidents after drinking are the commonest cause of death in young men, and one in three drivers killed in road accidents have blood alcohols over the legal limit. The number of innocent people killed each year by drivers with blood alcohol over the legal limit is 12,000. Even AT the legal limit, you are four times more likely to crash.

I hope Sal's shown this to Steve, seeing how he rides his motorcycle.

The long-term effects of alcohol are, among other things: damage to the liver due to inflammation and scarring, bleeding and ulcers in the stomach, cancer of the mouth and throat, brain damage, interference with your sex life, depression, psychiatric disorders, violence.

Wish Cilla would interfere with my sex life.

Drinking in pregnancy can also cause damage to the unborn child and it may be born very small, wizened, and brain damaged.
Women's bodies are more affected by alcohol than men's and therefore it does more damage to them.

I wonder if this is because men have more water in their bodies and therefore the drink would be more diluted than in women's?

Drinking in children—some of the facts that I could find:

—nine out of ten children try alcohol by the age of 14 and this is the same for boys and girls

—most of these try it at home

—children who smoke also try alcohol

—boys tend to drink beer and lager while girls prefer Martini and Advocat

—children who are keen on drinking alcohol are more influenced by their friends than by their parents

—boys and girls who drink a lot are seen by their friends as liking discos, going out a lot with friends, acting big and showing off, getting into trouble and fighting

—boys and girls who never drink are seen as the opposite

—children who drink a lot are seen as being more disliked by grown-ups than by other children, and those that don't drink at all are the opposite . . .

Can see why she got an 'A' for this. It went on for pages and pages, but I'd had enough.

Thursday 28th December
Today was OK. It snowed. I really like Cilla. Especially after she was so nice when I was drunk. Things are going well now. I hope she turns up at Sam's New Year's Eve party. Randy Jo's away!

Saturday 30th December
Holidays are great because of sleeping in. Sam's mum rang to talk to my mum about the party. She thinks everyone will arrive with bottles of booze, and Sam's dad says he's going to frisk everyone as they come in. Poor Sam. Dad and Mum asked us what we thought about drink at supper, but ended up as usual by telling us what THEY thought.

I said I didn't think it was right to go down to the pub every night like Nick's dad who has a huge beer belly, and I wouldn't want to turn out like the tramps who hang out down at the

shopping centre, clutching bottles of cider. I said I supposed it
was all right to have the odd drink now and then.

Sally said that she had had her first drink when she was 10.
Mum had given her a little white wine and she had pinched the
bottle and finished it in her bedroom. There wasn't all that
much left. After gulping it down she had felt giddy and as if her
head was going to fall off, and had had to lie down. She had
taken it because she had always been good and she wanted to
do something against the grain. This really shocked Mum, who
had had no idea that this had happened, but both Mum and
Dad had to admit that they got a 'bit merry' sometimes. (I
didn't tell them that I had seen Father Christmas a bit more
than 'merry'.)

Sal also said that when she'd been out of work after failing
her exams she'd felt really depressed and had gone down to the
pub a lot, even though she didn't have much money. Now that
she was working at the local hairdressers, and had decided to
retake some of her exams, she wasn't drinking nearly so much.

Monday 1st January
NEW YEAR'S DAY—FEEL TERRIFIC! Went to Sam's party with
Nick. Turned out we were both dreading it. Nick told me that
there are three kinds of parties. At brothel ones, the same
music goes on and on as everyone is so busy that no one wants
to get up to change it. At booze-ups, everyone drinks lager or
beer, it's mates only, and they all end up in the street—for fags
or worse and a throw-up. Worst of all is the school disco, with
teachers making fools of themselves trying to dance and
wearing 'trendy' clothes. No touching drink or each other at
this!

Nick said he was only going to have one drink this time. He'd
got smashed at the last party so as not to feel left out, and
had found his mouth telling people exactly what he thought of
them. He had done the worst thing possible, drunk cider, then
wine, then vodka, then beer. Even I could have told him to at
least stick to drinking ONE kind of alcohol. He'd ended up lying

down in the road with his mate, to see who died first. Sam's party was great. Terrific music, lots of food and, like Nick, I stuck to one drink and saw the New Year in HEAVY SNOGGING CILLA. After midnight things with Cilla got even BETTER. Hope this is a catching disease.

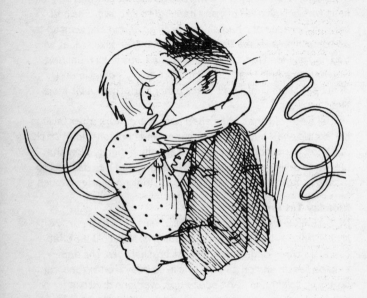

It makes me feel really Good.

INDEX

abnormal mobility and sprains 75–6
abuse, sexual 133–6
accidents and injuries 7–14
  fireworks 129–30
  in home 10, 12, 13–14, 17
  motorcyclists 9
  pedestrians 9
  sports and exercise 12, 13, 75–8
  see also road accidents
aches, *see* pain
acne, *see* spots and pimples
Acquired Immune Deficiency Syndrome,
  see AIDS
acupuncture 59
addiction 24–32
  see also drugs; smoking
advertisements, tobacco 67, 70
AIDS:
  causes 96, 97
  dangers of 95, 127
  and death 98
  prevention 94
  true and false about 99–100
alcohol, *see* drinking
allergies and allergens 58, 62, 79
ambulance 8
amphetamines 25, 26, 27, 30
ankle, sprained 75–6, 77
anorexia nervosa 104, 106
antibiotics 99
antibodies 58
antihistamines 59, 63
anus 115, 116, 118
anxiety about health 1–6
apocrine glands 116
appendicitis, fear of 67
appetite, loss of 23
arguing, *see* rows
arm, broken 10, 11, 78
armpits 42, 44, 116
asthma 77, 79–80
athlete's foot 119–20, 122
attractiveness 46

bacteria:
  and disease 97
  and smells 116
  and tooth decay 124–5
  balance and ear 82

balls 44, 118
bandages 82
basketball 78
bath as soporific 32
bedwetting 84
beer 148, 150
bikes, *see* cycling
bites, insect 89
blackheads 49, 53
blisters 130
blood:
  and allergies 58
  amount of 133
  bleeding gums 125
  nose bleed 14
  periods 33–40, 73
  sugar 27
  system, *see* heart
body odour (BO), *see* smells
bombykol 116
bone, broken 10, 11, 78
boobs, *see* breasts
boredom 46
bottling things up 21
brace, tooth 127
brain:
  bruising (concussion) 9, 11, 12
  damaged by drugs 29, 30
  heaviest recorded 132
  nerve cells in 133
  see also head
breasts:
  nipples 2, 116, 128
  size and development 35–6, 38
brown, getting 88
brushing teeth 124, 125–6
BSE (mad cow disease) 72, 92
bullying, *see* teasing and bullying
burns 86–8, 129–30
burping 115
butane gas sniffing 30, 31

calloguses 121
cancer:
  cervical 94
  lung, *see under* lung diseases
  throat and mouth (and alcohol) 149
cannabis 24, 25, 26, 27, 28–9
cap (contraceptive) 95–6

car:
   sickness 4, 82–3, 90–1
   see also road accidents
cerebral palsy 77
cervix 94, 96
chest infections 30, 79
cider 148
cigarettes, *see* smoking
cleanliness and hygiene 38, 50, 115–22
   teeth 124, 125–6
   see also smells
clinic 98, 100
cocaine 25, 27, 30
coitus interruptus 94
cold sore 99
collar bone broken 78
'coming', *see* ejaculation
compression and sprains 75–6
concentration loss and drugs 29
conception *see* contraception;
      pregnancy; reproduction
concussion 9, 11, 12
condoms 55, 93–4, 97, 99
confidentiality by doctor 131
contraception 55, 93–6
cooling body 117
corns 121
cough, smoker's 3, 66
crabs (pubic lice) 96, 97, 100
crack 30
cramps, *see* stomach aches and cramps
crash helmets 9, 10
creams and lotions:
   for bites 89
   for bottom 86
   in first aid kit 82
   for pierced ears 132
   for pubic lice 100
   for spots 50, 51, 52, 53
   for sunburn 87
   for verrucas 120
   see also pills and medicine
cycling 15, 16
   accidents 7–9, 10–11, 14
   and heart beat 3
   and weight loss 105

death:
   from AIDS 98
   from butane gas sniffing 30, 31
   from drowning 9, 119
   from drunk driving 149
   from ecstasy (drug) 30
   from heart attack 1

from road accidents 9
   from smoking 65, 66, 69
   suicide 22, 91
decay, tooth 124–5
deformity and sprains 75–6
dehydration 146
dentists 123–7
deodorants 116
depression:
   and alcohol 149
   and drugs 29, 30, 31
   and love 101
   and pain 76
   recognizing 22–3
   and unemployment 91
   and weather 85
   and weight 106
   see also moods
diabetes 27
diaphragm (contraceptive) 95–6
diarrhoea 24, 30, 38, 85–6
diets, *see* food; overweight people
disabled people 77
disease, *see* illness, disease and
      infection
divorce 20, 21, 22, 84, 88–9
dope, *see* cannabis
dreams, wet 47
drinking:
   alcohol 25, 144–52
   liquids in illness 86, 88
driving, *see* car; road accidents
drowning 9, 119
drugs 24–32
   and AIDS 100
   for curing illness, *see* creams and
      lotions; pills and medicine
   steroids and sport 77
   see also drinking; smoking
Durex 93
   see also condoms

ears:
   and balance 82
   lobe as erogenous zone 2
   pierced 127–8, 132
eating, *see* food
eccrine glands 117
ecstasy (drug) 30
eggs, *see* ovaries and eggs
ejaculation 47; 93
electrocution 13
elevation and sprains 75–6
emotions, *see* feelings

erection 44, 45
erogenous zones 2
ethyl alcohol 148
excretion 118, 133
exercise and sport:
  and accidents and injuries 12, 13,
    75–8
  amount per week 11
  and asthma 77, 79–80
  and heart 1, 3, 133
  need for 32
  sex as 54
  and weight loss 105
  see also cycling; running
eyes:
  glasses 138–43
  seeing double 11
  strain and television 4

face:
  makeup 49, 50
  see also ears; head; moustache;
    mouth; nose; spots and pimples
fallopian tubes 96
false teeth 127
farming: tobacco 91
farting 115, 118
fat, *see* weight
fed up, feeling, *see* moods
feelings:
  and asthma 79
  let out 15, 19–21
  repressed 21
  and sex 44, 46
  and sweating 117
  and unemployment 91
  see also depression; moods
feet problems 119–21, 122
fermentation 147
fertilization 47, 93
fighting, *see* rows
fillings 127
fireworks 129–30
first-aid kit 82
flasher 85
fleas, cat 89
flu 130
fluoride toothpaste 126
follicles, hair 50, 52
food and eating problems:
  basics of good diet 112
  and body smell 116
  calories 112–14
  eating before drinking 149

overeating 23, 30, 103; *see also*
  overweight
  questions about 110–11
  undereating 23, 104, 106; *see also*
  underweight
  unhealthy 3, 46
  vegetarianism 73
  weight-loss diets 105, 112–14
foot problems 119–21, 122
football 77–8
fractures 10, 11, 78
French letter, *see* condoms
friends:
  and drinking 150
  and drugs 28
  rows with 22
  and smoking 66
  suicide of 22
fungal infections 98, 119–20, 122

gas (butane) sniffing 30, 31
gay people 60–1, 99
germs 38
glands 39, 50, 52, 116, 117
glasses (spectacles) 138–43
glue sniffing 30, 31
gonorrhoea 96, 97–8
grass, *see* cannabis
growth:
  hormone deficiency 105
  and pituitary gland 39
  see also height; puberty; weight
gum disease 125

hair, body:
  chest 44
  development 35
  follicles and spots 50, 52
  moustache 5, 42
  pubic 42, 44
  underarm 42, 44
hand injured 78
hangover 146
'hard' drugs 24, 25, 27, 30
hash, *see* cannabis
hayfever 56–63
head:
  injuries 9, 11, 12, 13, 77
  see also brain; face; headaches
headaches:
  and concussion 11
  and depression 23
  from hangover 146
  and hayfever 57

headaches (*cont*.):
  migraines 131
  not to do with sight 143
  and television 4
  and temperature 130
  and tiredness 17
  worry about 16
heart:
  attack and disease 1, 91
  as pump 1, 3, 133
height:
  girls taller 44
  increase 44
  short people 42, 107–8, 109
  tall people 108–9
  and weight 103–4
helplessness 23, 91
hemp, *see* cannabis
hepatitis 128
heroin 24, 25, 27, 30
herpes 97, 98–9
high on drugs 25, 29
histamine 58
HIV 97, *see also* AIDS
holidays 15–16, 81–9
home:
  accidents in 10, 12, 13–14, 17
  running away from 23
homeopathy 59
homosexuality 60–1, 99
hopelessness 23
hormones:
  and boys 44
  and contraceptive pill 94–5
  growth, deficiency of 105
  and periods 37, 39
  and pregnancy 37
  and spots 50
hospital:
  after accident 10, 12–13
  visiting people in 37
hygiene, *see* cleanliness
hypnosis 6, 59
hypochondriasis 1–6

ice and sprains 75–6
illness, disease and infection:
  asthma 77, 79–80
  cerebral palsy 77
  chest infections 30, 79
  diarrhoea 24, 30, 38, 85–6
  and drugs: addictive 30, 31; healing,
    see pills and medicines
  and ear piercing 127–8

flu 130
fungal infections 98, 119–20, 122
hayfever 56–63
heart 1, 91
hepatitis 128
inherited 58
IUD and risk of infection 95
meningitis 45–6, 130
serious, depression and 22
and sex, *see* sexually transmitted
    diseases
and smoking 3, 68, 69
and swimming pools 119–22
  see also death; lung diseases; pain;
    sickness; viral illness
immunology 5
impotence 69
infection, *see* illness
influenza 130
inherited diseases 58
injections:
  of insulin for diabetes 27
  against measles 10
  against tetanus 8, 10
injuries, *see* accidents
insomnia:
  and depression 23
  and hot drink 54–5
  and noise 56
  pills for 16, 24
insulin 27
intra-uterine device, *see* IUD
isolation 23
IUD (intra-uterine device) 95

jabs, *see* injections
Johnny, *see* condoms

kidneys 30, 133
kissing 152
  record 123
  unsavoury grown-ups 4, 51, 65

lager 148, 150
late, staying out 16
law and drugs 27, 28, 29
laxatives 106
lice 96–7, 100
'life changes', *see* puberty
lighter-fuel sniffing 30, 31
liquids, *see* drinking
liver damage 30, 149
lockjaw, *see* tetanus
loneliness 22

long sight 142
lotions, *see* creams and lotions
love 44, 84
    see also sex
LSD 26, 27
lung diseases 91
    asthma 77, 79–80
    cancer, danger of 3, 69
lysergic acid (LSD) 26, 27

mad cow disease, *see* BSE
makeup and spots 49, 50
marijuana, *see* cannabis
marriage, *see* divorce; parents
masturbation 44, 47, 54, 97
mates, *see* friends
measles injection 10
medicines, *see* creams and lotions; pills
        and medicines
melanin and melanocytes 88
memory loss and drugs 29
meningitis 45–6, 130
menstruation 33–40, 73
mental problems 30, 149
    see also depression; moods; suicide
methyl alcohol 148
mind, *see* mental problems
moods 15–23, 46
    PMT 38
    see also depression
mosquito bites 89
moths 116
motion sickness 4, 82–3, 90–1
motorcyclists 9, 61
moustache 5
    shaving 42, 52, 143
mouth:
    cancer 149
    teeth 123–7
muscles, development of 44

nakedness 35, 57, 86, 138
natural method (contraception) 94–5
nerve cells in brain 133
nipples 2, 116
    pierced 128
no, saying 133–6
non-specific urethritis, *see* NSU
nose:
    bleed 14
    broken 12
    cocaine damage to 30
    pierced 132
NSU (non-specific urethritis) 97, 99

nudity 35, 57, 86, 138

odour, *see* smells
opticians and eye tests 139–43
oral contraceptives 55, 94–5
oral gratification 31
ovaries and eggs 37, 93, 94, 95
    fertilization 47, 93
overweight people:
    addiction to food 30
    examples of 102, 105–7
    and height 103–4
    losing weight 16, 23, 105, 112–14
ovulation 95

PAD (Pain, Abnormal mobility, Deformity)
        75–6
pain:
    and burns 130
    and crushed hand 78
    and depression 76
    self-healing 67–8
    and sprains 75–6
    treatment for, *see* paracetemol
    see also headaches; stomach aches
        and cramps
paracetemol 16, 27
    in first-aid kit 82
    for period pain 40
    for sore throat 45
    and sprained ankle 76
    and sunburn 87
    and temperature 130, 131
paranoia 30
parents:
    depressed 22
    and divorce 20, 21, 22, 84, 88–9
    and drugs 28
    expectations too high 22
    rows between 15, 19–20, 21, 84
parties 144–5, 150, 151
passive smoking 65, 66, 69
pedestrians and accidents 9
peers, *see* friends
penicillin 27, 98
penis:
    apocrine glands near 116
    erection 44, 45
    flashing 85
    size 44, 45
    warts 96–7, 98
    words for 118
periods 33–40, 73, 96
    and acne 52

periods (*cont.*):
  pains 37, 40, 132, 136
pheromones 116
piercing:
  ears 127–8, 132
  nipples 128
  nose 132
pills and medicine 27
  and asthma 80
  contraceptive 55, 94–5
  and hayfever 58–9, 62–3
  laxatives 106
  penicillin 27, 98
  sleeping 16, 24
  for STDs 98, 99
  and travel sickness 82–3, 90–1
  see also creams and lotion;
    paracetemol
pimples and spots 46, 49–53
pituitary gland and growth 39
plaque on teeth 125
plaster for broken bones 10, 11
plasters 82
PMT (pre-menstrual tension) 38
podiatrist 121
poisonous substances, *see* drinking;
    drugs; smoking
police drugs squad 27, 29, 31
pollen and hayfever 57, 58, 62, 63
pollution:
  and asthma 79
  from industry 91
  passive smoking 65, 66, 69
pot, *see* cannabis
pre-menstrual tension, *see* PMT
pregnancy:
  and alcohol 149
  danger of 55, 93
  and hormones 37
  prevention, *see* contraception
  and smoking 65
  see also reproduction
prick, *see* penis
prison for drug offences 27, 29
proof spirit 148
protectives, *see* condoms
puberty 4
  in boys 41–8
  in girls 33–40, 52, 73
  see also hair, body; spots
pubic hair 42, 44
pubic lice 96–7, 100
pus 97
pushers, drug 27

raves 30
rebellion and drugs 28
reproduction 43
  fertilization 47, 93
  see also pregnancy; sex
rest and sprains 75–6
rhythm method 94–5
RICE (Rest, Ice, Compression, Elevation)
    75–6
riding accident 12, 78
road accidents 7–12
  car 9, 149
  cycling 7–9, 10–11, 14
  and drinking 149
rows:
  between brothers and sisters 17–19
  between parents 15, 19–20, 21, 84
rubbers, *see* condoms
running 73, 74–5, 77, 79
  away 23
runs, *see* diarrhoea

salicylic acid 120, 122
sanitary towels 34–5, 36, 37
school:
  sex taught at 43
  staying away from 23, 129–37
  see also work at school
scratching 115
sea sickness 83
sebum and sebaceous glands 50, 52
seeing, *see* eyes
self-criticism 23
self-defence 136
sex 44–7
  age of first experiences 60
  and disease, *see* sexually transmitted
    diseases
  erogenous zones 2
  homosexuality 60–1, 99
  impotence 69
  masturbation 44, 47, 54
  pheromones 116
  pregnancy fear 55
  reproduction 43, 47
  sexual abuse 133–6
  survey 60
  taught at school 43
  see also contraception; puberty;
    reproduction
sexually transmitted diseases 92,
    96–100
  prevention 94, 96, 99, 100
shakes and drugs 30

shaving 42, 52, 143
sheaths, *see* condoms
sherry 148
shoes 121
short people 42, 107–8, 109
short sight 142
sickness (vomiting):
   and diarrhoea 86
   induced in attempt to lose weight 106
   motion 4, 82–3, 90–1
   words for 118
sight, *see* eyes
size, *see* height; weight
skating accident 13
skin:
   bacteria on 116
   sunburn 86–8
   sweat glands 117
   tests for allergies 62
   see also makeup; spots; sunburn
skunk (cannabis) 29
sleep:
   bath as soporific 32
   need for 4
   problems, *see* insomnia
smells 140
smells, bad 115–17, 123
   deodorants 116
   and smoking 65, 67, 68, 115
   of unsavoury grownups 4, 65
smoking 64–71
   advertisements 67, 70
   behind bike sheds 6
   and cancer 69
   by children, statistics of 70
   and coughing 3, 66
   and drinking 150
   and drugs 25, 29
   giving up 68, 70
   and heart 1
   land used to grow tobacco 91
   reasons for starting 65–7
   reward for never starting 69, 71
   stink of 65, 67, 68, 115
sneezing 56, 58, 61
sniffing:
   butane gas 30, 31
   glue 30, 31
   and hayfever 56, 61
soap 50, 52
solvent abuse 30, 31
special clinics 100
spectacles 138–43
speed, *see* amphetamines

spermatic cords 96
spermicides 96
sperms 37
   fertilizing eggs 47, 93
   numbers of 93
   vulnerable 44
spirits (alcohol) 148
spirochaete 97
sport, *see* exercise and sport
spots and pimples 46, 49–53
sprained ankle 75–6, 77
sprays for asthma 80
STDs, *see* sexually transmitted diseases
step-families 88
sterilization 96
stink, *see* smells, bad
stomach aches and cramps:
   and alcohol 149
   and depression 23
   and diarrhoea 30, 38, 85–6
   and drugs 30, 31
   and periods 37, 40, 132, 136
strangers, avoiding 134, 135–6
sugar:
   blood 27
   fattening 16
   and tooth decay 124–5, 126–7
suicide:
   attempts 91
   of friend 22
summer holidays 15–16, 81–9
sunburn 86–8
sunlight and spots 50
suppliers, drug 27
sweat 117
swimming:
   drowning 9, 119
   pools and infection 119–22
syphilis 97

tablets, *see* pills
talking about problems 22
tampons 35, 37, 40
tanning 88
tax from smokers 70
teasing and bullying:
   about body size 105, 106–8, 109
   about hayfever 61
   about wearing glasses 139
   avoiding 134–5
   in family 73–4
teeth care 123–7
television 4, 142
temperature, body 116–17, 130, 131–2

testicles 44, 118
tetanus injection 8, 10
THC (tetrahydrocannabinols) 28
thighs 2
thin people 106–7
Third World agriculture 91
throat:
    cancer 149
    sore 45
thrush 97, 98
tiredness 17, 23, 30
tobacco, *see* smoking
toilet, *see* excretion
tooth care 123–7
toothpaste 126
tummy, *see* stomach

ulcers 149
underweight people 104, 106–7
unemployment 91, 92
unhappiness, *see* depression; moods
uppers, *see* amphetamines
urethritis 97, 99
uterus 37

vagina:
    and diaphragm (cap) 95
    discharge 37, 97
    warts 96, 98–9
    words for 118
vegetarianism 73
verrucas 120, 121, 122
violence 4, 149
viral illness 45–6, 97–8, 130
    and swimming pools 119, 120–1, 122
vision, *see* eyes
vocal chords 44

voice breaking 41, 44
vomiting, *see* sickness

walking: pedestrians and accidents 9
wanking, *see* masturbation
war 91–2
warts 120–1, 122
    penile and vaginal 96–7, 98
washing, *see* cleanliness
weather:
    and asthma 79
    and depression 85
weight 102–7
    and height 103–4
    see also overweight; underweight
wetting bed 84
wheelchair 77
whisky 148
wind, breaking 115, 118
wine 147
withdrawal method 94
womb, 95, *see also* uterus
words for parts of body 118
work at school:
    good marks for 92
    and hayfever 58
    homework diary 90
    planning 101
    problems and depression 22, 23
    tests and exams 58, 136–7
    see also school

x-rays 9

youngest, being 74

zits 46, 49–53